The Wall Street Diet

The Wall Street Diet

The Surprisingly Simple Weight Loss Plan for
Hardworking People Who Don't Have Time to Diet

Heather Bauer, RD,CDN,
and Kathy Matthews

HYPERION

NEW YORK

This book is intended as a reference volume only, not a medical manual. The information contained herein is designed to help you make informed decisions about your health and your weight; it is not intended as a substitute for any treatment that may have been prescribed by your doctor or health care professional. If you suspect that you suffer from a medical condition, we urge you to seek advice and guidance from a health care professional.

The mention of specific companies and organizations listed in this book does not imply endorsement by the publisher, nor does mention of specific companies, organizations, or authorities imply that they endorse this book.

The contact information for companies, organizations, and websites listed in this book were correct at time of publication.

Library of Congress Cataloging-in-Publication Data

Bauer, Heather.
    The Wall Street diet : the surprisingly simple weight loss plan for hardworking people who don't have time to diet / Heather Bauer and Kathy Matthews.
        p. cm.
    Includes bibliographical references and index.
    ISBN 978-1-4013-2258-8 (alk. paper)
    1. Businesspeople—Nutrition. 2. Executives—Nutrition. 3. Reducing diets.
4. Weight loss. I. Matthews, Kathy. II. Title.
    RA777.63.B38 2008
    613.2'5—dc22   2008001875

Hyperion books are available for special promotions, premiums, or corporate training. For details contact Michael Rentas, Proprietary Markets, Hyperion, 77 West 66th Street, 12th floor, New York, New York 10023, or call 212-456-0133.

Book design by Richard Oriolo

FIRST EDITION

10 9 8 7 6 5 4 3 2 1

To my parents, Beth and Nathan Greenbaum, for always believing in me. And to my incredibly supportive, motivating, and endlessly loving husband and best friend, Ross. And finally, joyously, to my beautiful daughter, Zander Reese Bauer.

H.B.

Contents

Acknowledgments

T he *Wall Street Diet* has been an incredible journey and one that I could not have successfully completed without the help of some very smart, generous, and talented people.

I am endlessly grateful to my agent, Margret McBride, for sticking with me through the long gestation of this book and for introducing me to the wonderful and brilliant Kathy Matthews. And thanks to Kim McBride for her clever suggestions.

Judy and Joel Bauer, my incredibly loving in-laws, got the ball rolling by introducing me to Margret McBride. They've always been my most enthusiastic supporters.

My great thanks to Kathy Matthews for her ability to hear my voice and understand my ideas and translate them into written words. That ability is truly a gift. I am so glad to have met her, not only because of this project, but also because I've found a wonderful and supportive friend. Her calm demeanor and incredible writing skills, combined with her sense of humor, make her a true pro.

I am so grateful to the team at Hyperion. They have all been a dream to work with. Brenda Copeland, my editor, has from the very beginning shown an enthusiasm and zest for this book that is more than I could have ever asked for. I'm especially thankful to Will Schwalbe, Will Balliett, Ellen Archer, and Kathleen Carr, who supported this book from the very start. My thanks, too, to many others on the Hyperion team, including Beth Gebhard, Jane Comins, Navorn Johnson, Claire McKean, and Fritz Metsch.

My Nu-Train team is the world's greatest. I owe them all a debt of gratitude for their enthusiasm and support. Lauren Cutrona runs the show and is a wonderful and energetic presence. Stephanie Middleberg is always ready with a helping hand. And Molly Kyle has shown herself to be Nu-Train's greatest intern ever. Many thanks to you all.

I must acknowledge my brother, Jordan, and my sister, Jessica, for always pushing me to work harder. My loving and wonderful grandmother Mimi Nickelsporn, your constant check-ins always mean the world to me. And to the rest of my family and friends, thank you for your support and encouragement.

And finally, I must thank my fantastic clients. You all inspired me to create the Wall Street Diet. Your stories and your successes make each day special for me. Thank you for your inspiration. Keep eating well!

Heather Bauer

This book has been an extraordinary voyage. Heather Bauer is the real deal: smart, perceptive, funny, energetic, and an absolute delight to work with. Her clients know how lucky they are to have her, and her dedication to them is remarkable. It was my good fortune to be able to participate in this project with her.

Margret McBride, our agent, has been the dynamic force who championed this book from the beginning, and to her and her office staff, particularly Faye Atchison, many, many thanks.

Working with Brenda Copeland, our editor at Hyperion, has been a joy. Her enthusiasm and total dedication to this project have been nothing short of awe-inspiring. Her sense of humor in particular has smoothed the road and turned Wall Street into Easy Street. I add my thanks to the team at Hyperion mentioned by Heather. They've been truly extraordinary in their willingness to go the limit for this book.

On a personal note, I must once again apologize to my family for yet another year of occasional neglect. Fred, Greg, and Ted, you have, as always, been my anchors and my inspiration. Thanks also to the Island Girls, Jean Drumm, Julie Karpeh, and particularly Nancy Nolan, for giving me a place to work and not making me go to the beach.

Kathy Matthews

The Wall Street Diet

Introduction:
Welcome to Wall Street

You can see them hailing a taxi at 5:30 A.M. on Park Avenue or rushing to catch the 6:10 from Greenwich to Grand Central Station. They're bankers, lawyers, CEOs, CFOs—successful, hardworking people who are at the top of their field and the top of their game—and they're heading to Wall Street. They're ambitious, of course, and the determined looks on the faces of these men and women would convince you that they could accomplish almost anything. And they can. They close deals, manage billions, hire and fire. When it comes to work, they've got the world on a string. But the one thing they've had trouble figuring out is how to lose weight. It's not for lack of intelligence or effort. It's not for lack of drive or focus, and it's certainly not because they don't understand nutrition. Some of them know nearly as much about weight loss as I do, since they've been on every diet you've ever heard of—and some you haven't. So why have these otherwise successful people struggled with their weight? It's a four-letter-word: work.

For the Wall Street elite, the elephant in the room that no one has addressed before—certainly no diet—is their work: they work long hours, entertain frequently, and travel too much. Their work dominates their lives and they're not interested in changing that. Some of them never cook, rarely shop, and have little time for an exercise regime. They want to continue to entertain business associates, work long hours, and drink a glass of wine while losing weight and maintaining their overall health.

These people came to see me as a last resort. A doctor or a friend had told them that I was a nutritionist who was different. They'd already heard that I wouldn't hand them a sheet of menus. This clientele offered a special challenge when it came to weight loss. They weren't going to count points, cook special meals, order off "diet" menus, or give up too much of what they enjoyed when it came to dining out. They simply weren't interested in making what they eat a very high priority in their day. Many of them had tried other weight loss plans and found themselves frustrated and annoyed by the demands of these plans and the results they experienced. Of *course* they could lose weight if they could portion off part of their day to shop, measure, and cook. But they couldn't and they wouldn't.

This was the challenge I faced in constructing the Wall Street Diet: devise an effective weight loss plan that could fit seamlessly into a busy, demanding, hard-charging lifestyle. It had to be nutritionally sound, safe of course, and highly effective. It had to be simple to understand— no complicated categories or combinations—and it had to be totally portable. It had to work in the airport, at the highway rest stop, and at the Ritz in Paris. It had to be bulletproof when it came to buffets, cocktail parties, and lazy Sunday afternoons at home. In other words, these people needed a simple plan that started with *them*. Their lifestyle wasn't going to change. They couldn't work with a diet that asked them to revise their lives; they needed a diet that revised the very concept of what a diet is. That was the key for me. Don't start with the diet: start with the lifestyle.

Here are the obstacles that make weight loss such a challenge for the men and women of Wall Street:

- They have no time (to cook; to shop; to make food a priority in their lives).

- They endure business meetings and conferences where the only food choices are high in fat, carbs, and calories. (Bagel or giant muffin?)

- They entertain frequently and struggle with tempting menu choices.

- They face daunting travel itineraries that limit their food options: What do you eat at the airport? How do you resist the hotel breakfast buffet?

- They have a personal life that includes dining out, brunches with friends, and family meals that don't often promote weight loss goals.

- They have a business image to maintain. (They have no interest in making their private struggles with weight and diet a public issue among colleagues and clients.)

- They have no patience for long-term projects. (They are driven to tick things off their lists and move on. For them slow results = no results.)

The Wall Street Diet is the diet that works. It provides a framework of simple but powerful strategies and suggestions—a business plan for effective weight loss—that speaks to time-starved, pressured people who are looking for real results. It addresses real-life obstacles and gives specific, proactive ways to gain control over situations that in the past spelled diet disaster. *The Wall Street Diet* will train you to develop a skill set that most failed dieters need but have never addressed. The focus is not just emphasizing the right foods in the right amounts like most popular diets. Rather *The Wall Street Diet* walks readers through the process of developing a new approach to integrating improved food choices into a busy and often distracting schedule.

The Wall Street Diet is the first diet geared specifically to a very particular culture of hardworking people, and it's successful because it makes losing weight a seamless part of the corporate lifestyle rather than an add-on project to an already full schedule.

The Wall Street Diet Executive Summary

The Wall Street Diet is a unique approach to weight loss, which I can best describe by outlining the main tenets of my program. Here are the three critical issues—Power Points—that the Wall Street Diet confronts and conquers. They are the principles that inspire all of the effective weight loss strategies that inform this program:

Prioritize!

Setting priorities may sound familiar as a weight loss tool but the Wall Street Diet approach to weight control is unique. It's not about acknowledging that losing weight is important to you. That's a given. *The critical priority is recognizing how your lifestyle is standing in your way.* It's about appreciating the aspects of a demanding career that make weight control difficult, and devising strategies that help you avoid the pitfalls that you face every day. I've defined six catalysts to overeating. Many of these catalysts are generally unrecognized by my clients, who are, therefore, powerless to cope with them. Once you recognize these pitfalls, you can make conscious decisions about how you're going to handle them in the future. Instead of stumbling over food issues and letting situations dictate your responses, you can take control of eating habits and reach your goals.

The first step my clients make in prioritizing is examining the situations they face every day—some surprisingly remote from "eating" or "dieting"—that encourage them to lose their focus on eating healthfully. Sometimes just recognizing these pitfalls is half the battle.

Here's an example that is a "hidden" but *extremely* important issue for almost every single one of my clients: *free food!* Free food can cloud the priorities of all but the most focused. What happens to us when food is free? Whether you're a CEO in business class on an international flight facing a roster of food and drink choices meant to distract you from your uncomfortable seat, or a Whole Foods shopper passing the tray of cheese samples, your willpower dissolves. It is all too easy to persuade ourselves that if it's free, it doesn't count! This would not be an important issue if your only temptation was an occasional ham spread appetizer in the aisles of Costco. But when you're facing a minibar filled with Toblerone chocolates, giant Twix bars, and "gourmet" nut mixes, or an expense account dinner at a five-star restaurant with a stunning dessert cart, your mind may scream "No," but your corporate credit card and your taste buds rise up in an insistent chorus of "Yes!"

Free food is a huge pitfall, but not if you prioritize in advance. Simply recognizing your response to free food helps you to move from autopilot mode to something more proactive and effective.

Prepare!

What you eat each day is a choice, but it often doesn't seem that way. While researchers tell us that we make well over two hundred food choices daily, for my clients "choice" is not the operative word. For high-pressure, stressed-out corporate types, the vast majority of food decisions are made under less-than-ideal conditions. In fact, many of my clients tell me that they make only a handful of food-related decisions each week that are *not* influenced by work situations. They are rarely standing in their kitchens, searching their refrigerators for an appropriate, healthy, low-calorie meal. Rather they are shouting an order for a take-out lunch to someone who's making a food run from the office. Or they are jogging through an airport, having skipped breakfast, realizing that if they don't grab something in the next ten minutes, they'll have nothing to eat for the next six hours. You simply cannot survive these situations, and lose weight, without preparation. You need simple strategies to help you manage the onslaught of food decisions that threaten your waistline and your health.

> *If you think you can't lose weight because you don't have enough willpower, I have the solution. Preparation trumps willpower. If you are prepared for a "diet challenge," you don't need willpower!*

Two of the common issues faced by my clients that demand preparation are "force feeding" and social pressure.

"*Force feeding*" refers to the countless instances where my clients find themselves in situations analogous to that of a lab rat: situations in which they are pressured to make food choices that they would never make of their own volition. If you have ever sat at an all-day meeting that commenced with bagels and Danish, broke for a lunch of three choices of fatty sandwiches and cookies, and ended at 4 P.M. with coffee and brownies, you know that the "make healthy food choices" guidelines provided by popular diets are a virtually meaningless suggestion. The Wall Street Diet helps you manage force feeding and turn the tables on food service tyranny.

Social pressure is a huge, if generally unrecognized, pitfall for dieters in corporate positions. Travel and business meals put Wall Streeters in situations where they are not only powerless to dictate what foods they'd prefer but also pressured to choose foods that are unhealthy. I have heard countless stories of clients at convention gatherings or business meals who were shouted down when they tried to order healthy foods or skip alcoholic drinks. There's also the embarrassment factor: few people in a business situation want to make their diet a public issue. One woman told me that she tried to order what she thought was a healthy business dinner one evening, but the list of special requests that she gave the waiter when she ordered still lives in legend among her colleagues.

How do you handle both force feeding and social pressure? I provide simple but detailed strategies for handling these situations so you can cope gracefully and so that your food choices (or refusals) become invisible to your colleagues. As I tell my clients: preparation = moderation!

> *Prepare for the major "pressure points" in a business meal: alcohol and dessert. If you have strategies for dealing with these diet deal-breakers, you will succeed.*

Recover

Any business experiences economic fluctuations. The real test over time is how that business survives when it hits a rough patch. If survival is the game, recovery strategies are critical. And recovery is an essential aspect of the Wall Street Diet. Indeed, effective recovery is what turns a "diet" into a "lifestyle." I recall the client who told me, with more than a little challenge in his voice, how he met with colleagues in a Middle Eastern country where long meals were de rigueur and refusal of food was considered rude. "So," he asked, "what the heck was I supposed to do?" "Enjoy the food, have an effective meeting, and eat light the next day!" I told him. *You must accept and embrace the notion that* nothing *is a diet-breaker.* This seems to be particularly difficult for my female clients, who tend to link their diet success with personal worth. It's interesting (and the topic of another book!) how hard many of these women are on themselves when they make missteps in their diets. That's why it's critical for everyone—men and women alike—to recognize that knowing how to get back on track may be the single most important strategy of the Wall Street Diet.

"I lost forty pounds with Heather and I'll never be heavy again. Unlike other plans that teach you how to diet, she teaches you how to eat so that you lose weight and keep it off without any crazy restrictions. I eat out, I order in, I live my life!"
—SUSAN F., VICE PRESIDENT, INTERNATIONAL ADVERTISING COMPANY

While it's important to make a psychological recovery from an eating lapse—and I provide tips on how clients should think about their relative success and missteps—I have found that a concrete, *active* plan of recovery is far more effective than mental gymnastics alone. It's especially true for my highly focused, action-oriented clients. For that reason, I have a few simple and elegant recovery techniques that have proven effective.

Losing Weight Is Personal

It's about you and how you live and how you want to live. If you've tried and failed to lose weight in the past, you may feel discouraged. You may feel that it's the one thing you can't master. I'd like to introduce you to a few of my clients because you may find that their challenges match some of your own. They may be the inspiration that you need.

Susannah P.* is the CEO of a large and highly successful consulting company.

I had been having problems with my knees and my orthopedist told me that my body weight "exceeded my physical design capacity." As a former scientist, this resonated with me. I realized that I had to get serious about losing weight. I'd been so engrossed in my work and spent so many hours at the office that, frankly, I'd neglected myself. A friend who'd recently lost weight told me about Heather and so I went to see her. I had tried plenty of diets in the past but never very successfully, so it was hard to imagine what I could learn that would make the difference this time. But my friend was so enthusiastic I thought it would be worth a try. Heather's plan was an eye-opener for me because it was more of a *shift* than a regime. I'm methodical in my work and I resisted being methodical in my personal life. With Heather's diet, I didn't have to be. I didn't change anything about my lifestyle: I just learned how to manage to eat better by making wiser, more educated choices. Heather's snacks made a surprising difference. Now I always travel with Fiber Rich crackers,** and I always get an extra search at customs when I check off the box indicating that I'm bringing food into the country. But it's worth it because I've lost thirty pounds and my knees are fine now. I'm forever grateful to Heather because she changed my life.

Tom Z. is one of New York's top defense attorneys and a distinguished law professor.

My doctor sent me to Heather. He said it was lose weight or medicate! I'd never been on a diet before. I had no interest in learning anything about dieting or paying any special attention to what I ate. But I had to

* While based on real-life clients and their stories, some of the names and identities of people in this book have been obscured to preserve their privacy.
** A Wall Street Diet favorite snack.

admit that even the first class seats on British Air were starting to seem a little snug. I travel all the time. I eat out more than I eat at home. I guess that's why I've put on so much weight in the last few years. Heather talked to me about my lifestyle. She learned what I was unwilling to give up, such as wine, and what I could manage to live without. That was five years and sixty pounds ago. I had to make the hard decision that it was important to me to lose weight. But once I decided that, Heather made it easy. Now I can eat well anywhere in the world. If I can live the way I live and follow Heather's diet, anyone can.

And one more. Laura D. is a highly sought-after designer who splits her time between New York, Spain, and Hong Kong.

I've been on too many diets to think about, and they all were successful, but never for more than a month or so. I frankly resent having to think about what I eat as a punishment. I love to eat. I love restaurant life, and my work requires that I eat out constantly. But I got to the point where I was feeling uncomfortable in my skin. My clothes were tight even when I wore my "fat" clothes. I meet new people all the time and the way I look is important to me for all the usual reasons, but also because in my work it's critical that I make a good first impression. I needed help. Heather was a miracle for me. When I first saw her, I was following what I thought of as a "modified South Beach." She cleared my head about what I needed to eat and made it simple. I've lost twenty-two pounds, but here's the important part: I lost it six years ago! It's still lost! When a pound or two creeps back, I pay a little more attention and I'm back on track. My "fat" clothes are gone. I'll never need them again.

Much More Than Just a Numbers Game . . .

I'm proud of all my clients. Perhaps what I'm proudest of is that they manage to keep the weight off. I tell them, "The door is always open. I'd love to see you back if you need me." Some continue to see me on a regular basis. Some just send a holiday card and let me know they're doing well. Many get in touch now and again if they have a particular issue. And here's something that I've noticed in the years I've spent with these highly successful, hardworking people: weight is not just a number on the scale. It's got a lot to do with how you feel about yourself and your place in the world. And, honestly, I'm as concerned about this issue as about a number on the scale. When people lose weight, they tell me they're more successful. They feel empowered, stronger. The shy person can disappear and become more outgoing, outspoken. One client told me that since she lost weight, she's quicker to speak up at meetings and even to call out a colleague who's behaving badly. "No more wallpaper" is how she put it.

Weight loss can mean change. Be prepared. Clients tell me that when they lose weight they feel more clarity. Overweight is a cloud that hangs over so many aspects of your life. When the cloud dissipates, you see things that were previously obscured. Sometimes that vision moves you to do something different, something new. I've seen clients change jobs and even careers once they lost weight. Things that seemed closed to them suddenly opened. I had a lawyer who went back to school to begin a medical career. On a smaller scale, I've seen countless clients find free time, become more organized, join book clubs, start biking. It's all about how you feel. When you're eating poorly, you feel poorly and you feel bad about yourself. When you clear the debris of a bad diet, you take charge. It's amazing that it can all start with a Fiber Rich cracker and a mini cheese!

Eat Right Now!

If you're like most of my clients, you're thinking, "Well, this sounds great but it's a bad time to start because . . ." You can fill in the blank: "I've got a trip in two days." "I've got a wedding this weekend." "I'm heading into sales conference and things are crazy." So here's what I tell my clients: Now is a *perfect* time to start! Not tomorrow. Not next week. Not next month. Not the beginning of next quarter or the beginning of next year. Now! Start at your next meal. Start at the airport. Start when you get home from work today. Just start.

Commit to the Wall Street Diet and get started!
Commit to yourself.

Let me know how you're doing. I'm rooting for you. You can reach me at *www.WallStreetDiet.com.*

PART ONE

The Wall Street Diet
Begins with You

How It Began

I first began to work with my Wall Street warriors when I was the nutrition consultant at the Equinox Health Club at Broadway and Fiftieth Street in Manhattan. This club offered corporate membership plans to countless companies in the neighborhood, including Lehman Brothers, Morgan Stanley, and Cravath, Swaine & Moore. It was immediately apparent to me that my Equinox clientele existed in a different nutritional world from the people I had counseled in my previous job at Maimonides Medical Center in New York. The latter simply needed basic nutrition information about optimum food choices. The harried Equinox clients, on the other hand, needed to learn what to eat when they felt they had *no* choices. Their nutritional knowledge was generally impressive but their actual real-life habits were almost shocking. They rushed from meeting to meeting, skipped meals frequently, and grabbed giant cinnamon buns at the airport. (They were starving! They had no time! There was nothing else!)

Many of the Equinox patrons met with me because they were taking advantage of a membership freebie—a consultation with a nutritionist. Some of the people were truly interested in changing their eating patterns and losing weight; others were simply taking advantage of a corporate freebie. I quickly learned that I had to move very fast with this crowd. I basically had thirty minutes to convince them that they could eat better and lose weight if that was their goal. The truth was that most of them were not really interested in long-term results. They wanted something to happen ASAP. If their belts didn't feel looser in a few days, they'd move on and forget about it. And they had no patience for anything too complicated. There was no point in handing them sheets of printed menus or healthy recipes. There was no point in counting on them to change their daily routines. They weren't going to change their daily routines. They quite simply couldn't.

They were overworked, stressed out, and exhausted, and they didn't have any interest in spending extra time at the gym or in the kitchen. They didn't take time for themselves, and any time they had left over after work went to their families and friends. They weren't about to skip a soccer game with their kids or a girls' night out or a Mets game—rare treats—to make special meals. In fact, a common problem was that some of these people ate two dinners: one with clients and one "snack" dinner when they got home, exhausted, or, on the rare occasions when they got home early, one with their kids and another, later "adult" dinner.

Ultimately I came to realize that, in their secret hearts, most of my corporate clients believed that they'd take care of their health some glorious day in the future when they retired! But in the meantime they'd hit the wall: either a doctor or a spouse had told them they simply had to take care of themselves. (One of my thirty-eight-year-old clients was shocked to learn from her doctor that she had the cardiovascular health of an unhealthy old man as evidenced by her lipid levels and her blood pressure.) These people also complained that they just didn't feel well. They were often tired and irritable. They sometimes had difficulty concentrating. Their clothes were tight. And they felt out of control.

What quickly became obvious to me was that I couldn't start with a diet—my diet or any diet. Rather, I had to work backward beginning with my clients' challenges. Because the simple truth is that most diet books are based on the premise that overweight is a "food choice" problem. But I quickly realized that for many people—certainly for my clients—overweight is a "lifestyle" problem. The bottom line is that for time-pressured, high-powered, hardworking, type-A people, losing weight is not primarily about food choices at all; *it's about strategy*. Once I fully appreciated that, I spent my time with clients getting to know their challenges and "nonnegotiables."

Over time I developed a template that worked for these individuals. I created a reeducation program that helped them gradually transform their relationship to food. I gave them a simple outline of what they should be eating. I had them move slowly and adopt simple strategies bit by bit. I found foolproof ways to help them solve all their eating dilemmas, from high-calorie restaurant food to finding a healthy breakfast at the airport at 6 A.M. They began to feel physically better. They began to lose weight and to feel optimistic and in control of their health. The change was often dramatic.

Eventually I agreed to take on the job of nutrition consultant at the brand-new Equinox branch down on Wall Street in addition to my work at the midtown branch. The clientele was similar—bankers, traders, lawyers, CEOs, entrepreneurs—but by then I had an arsenal of effective strategies that I used to help my clients gain mastery over their eating challenges. I found that encouraging clients to develop their own personal blueprints for success was infinitely more effective than simply dictating food choices. These people were smart and they were results-driven: they needed to acknowledge that effective weight loss demands a flexible, personal strategy, and they needed support in implementing their particular strategies. Those strategies and supports are the heart of the Wall Street Diet.

I now have my own growing private practice. But I'm still working with the same type of clientele. They send their friends, and they send *their* friends. They tell others about my diet and insist that it's the only way they ever could have lost weight. And now it's your turn to try the Wall Street Diet.

Not a titan of Wall Street? You may not be a major deal maker, but you may well struggle with the same weight control issues that bring people to the Wall Street Diet.

- If you live a busy, stressful, demanding life,

- if weight loss is a high priority for you but following a diet is not,

- if you rush from commitment to commitment, squeezing in meals as you go,

- if you struggle to make the right food choices in situations that are challenging, or

- if you can't manage to fit your lifestyle to any existing diet,

you will find that the Wall Street Diet works as well on Main Street as it does in the heart of the financial district and that the strategies in this book will be your springboard to a new, slimmer future.

Your Wall Street Portfolio: What's Your Personal Eating ID?

You're smart. You're ambitious. You work hard and can accomplish almost anything you set your mind to. Why is losing weight such a challenge? It's old news that we're witnessing an obesity epidemic. The important and very personal news for you is that you caught it at the office: you've gained weight because along with your job comes too much heavy food and not enough light, healthy food. When you're not entertaining or working through lunch, you're trying to cram in appointments or errands. You're in a hurry and you want to grab something fast. But that often means too much fat, too many calories. Too often, you're victimized by your schedule when it comes to food. Too often, what you eat is not at all up to you, and too often, it's not what you prefer. You are, in effect, force-fed in countless unavoidable, even if often enjoyable, situations. No wonder you've struggled with weight.

But you're clever and energetic. You've got discipline and focus. You've set business goals and met them. You've wowed clients. You've structured deals and you've never had a problem keeping your eye on the bottom line. So let's look at how you can turn the skills you already possess to your own bottom line.

A workable plan is the first step to success. It's true in business; it's true in life. With the Wall Street strategies, you'll see that you don't need to keep making the same decisions about food. You can break through to the next level and send your personal stock soaring.

Take a look in the mirror. You're seeing your own best client. But how well do you know that client? You'd never approach a business prospect without researching them. You'd be fully versed in their company profile, their products and services, their strengths and weaknesses. It's time to turn that laser focus on yourself, because just as research is the basis for success in business, so it's going to be for your diet success. The Wall Street Diet is going to guide you to a new business plan when it comes to food.

What kind of eater are you? What are your particular eating challenges? The people I work with have one thing in common—a demanding job that limits their time and dominates their lives. But they have many differences. Some cook; some don't. Some like to enjoy a glass of wine or a glass of scotch, while others demand at least two daily cups of coffee. Some do the family shopping; some rarely buy food and only order in or eat out. Some travel constantly; some rarely. Some have families; some are single. Of course, they all have different food likes and dislikes. In my ten years as a nutritionist I've come to realize that the only common denominator among my clients is the need for a personalized plan, something that is going to build on their strengths while taking into account their challenges. I found out quickly that my clients were not going to lose weight by "learning" my diet (or any diet for that matter), which is why I make a point of "learning" them. My approach—the Wall Street approach—is to help my clients develop an eating plan that suits their lifestyle and taste. With a personalized diet there's less to remember and a much better chance of long-term success. Of course the Wall Street Diet is already highly personalized for people with a busy work life, but let's do this right and fine-tune the diet to your particular needs. You'll see that by taking a look at just a few issues that affect your eating patterns and choices, you'll get yourself one step closer to weight loss success.

"I've been on quite a number of diets before. I'd always start out with great enthusiasm and then I'd find myself in a few situations where I simply couldn't follow the diet and so I'd go off it, give up and feel like a failure. Work is a big part of my life and that was always a problem with other diets. Not the Wall Street Diet. The best thing about Heather's diet is that she didn't start with a plan I needed to follow; she started with me. She found out how I like to eat, how often I eat out, what my life is really like. And then she fit the plan to me. For example, I'm definitely a Clean Plate Club Eater. I never saw a diet that dealt with this aspect of my eating personality. But those tips really helped me. And I've been on the Wall Street Diet ever since. I've lost forty-one pounds and kept them off for four years. It's not really a diet for me anymore. It's just how I eat."

—BARBARA G., PORTFOLIO MANAGER, INVESTMENT FIRM

The Nonnegotiables

When I began working with my Wall Street clients, it quickly became apparent that almost all of them had nonnegotiables. Remember, these people are used to wheeling and dealing. Their impulse is to negotiate for what they want, and they have clear ideas on what constitutes a deal breaker. For some of them, the nonnegotiable was pasta; for others it was their daily orange juice, a second cup of coffee, or a diet soda. One client said that he couldn't survive without his evening Jack Daniel's. There was no point in telling these people that they had to eliminate the cherished bits of their daily diet that made life a pleasure for them. I knew that if I even tried, I'd never see them again. So I learned to love nonnegotiables, and to help my clients learn how to manage them.

If you want to lose weight, you have to make choices. And you can't have everything you want, at least not all the time. We accept this reality in just about every other part of life, but many of us have trouble accepting it when it comes to food. Of course, not everyone has a nonnegotiable, and some people are willing to give up certain pleasures for quicker weight loss. But in general, I've found that when people understand that they can retain the pleasure that food and drink give them—as long as they learn to thoughtfully manage these nonnegotiables—they're well on their way to a new, slimmer lifestyle that will be permanent.

So how do you manage nonnegotiables? You have to be selective and limit your intake. My Jack Daniel's client still, three years later, enjoys his JD in the evening and maintains his weight loss. But he's very careful about his carb intake and he's learned how to eat well while he travels.

When you get to The Plan in Part II, you'll see how you can incorporate alcohol, dessert, pasta—almost anything you really enjoy—into your diet. (Of course there are deal breakers: a bag of Doritos or a pint of Ben & Jerry's ice cream won't ever fit into your diet. You have to be realistic about your choices and always try to opt for the healthy one.) Once you've made a commitment to work toward your weight loss goal, you can identify your nonnegotiable and work it into *your* plan.

The Great Eating Divide: Clean Plate vs. Controlled

Yin or yang? Male or female? Regular or decaf? As I began to work with hardworking, stressed-out clients, it quickly became apparent that most of them fell into one of two groupings that I identified over time and through trial and error: Clean Plate Club Eaters or Controlled Eaters. I could usually ascertain where a client fell within a few minutes and with only a few questions. In fact, many of the Clean Plate Club Eaters would identify *themselves*: I'd simply ask "Are you a Clean Plate Club Eater?" and they'd either give me a puzzled look (which meant no) or they'd answer with an emphatic yes. In simplest terms, a Clean Plate Club Eater will eat everything on the plate; a Controlled Eater will stop when full.

Determining which of these two groups you belong to is important. No one diet suits everyone, but this defining category will allow you to address weaknesses and capitalize on strengths common to your personal eating style. The truth is that while most diets ask you to change temporarily in order to lose weight, you're always going to go back to being you. People fail at diets because while they may be able to temporarily change what they eat while they're on a particular diet, eventually they revert to their own comfortable eating habits. But once you recognize that you *are* a certain type of eater, you can tweak the Wall Street Diet so that it suits you and guarantees you success. Not for six weeks or six months, but forever. This approach has been remarkably successful with my clients and I know it will be for you, too. You'll discover that certain of my guidelines are geared for Clean Plate Club Eaters (CPCers), while others are for Controlled Eaters (CEs). Of course these groupings are not totally exclusive and there is sometimes some overlap. But almost all the clients I've worked with have been able to quickly recognize their category, which in turn helps us to deal with their strengths and weaknesses.

Read through the questions to see which group you belong to:

Are You a Clean Plate Club Eater?

- **Do you generally eat everything on your plate?**

- **Do you pick off others' plates?**

- **Are you a fast eater?**

- **Do you have trigger foods—like sugar, salt, or bread, or even cheese or nuts—that can prompt a binge?**

- **Do you sneak food?**

- **Do you hit the bread basket with gusto when you eat out?**

- **Do you tend to lose weight on vacation?**

- **Do you tend to eat more when you're alone?**

- **Is it especially hard for you to control your eating at night?**

- **When it comes to snack foods like chips, is an open bag an empty bag for you?**

- **Are you a poor water drinker?**

- **Are buffets a real challenge for you?**

- **Are you a Veteran Dieter?**

Are You a Controlled Eater?

- **Do you stop eating when full?**

- **Can you take one piece of bread from the bread basket?**

- **Can you take a single cookie from a platter, or can you be satisfied with a handful of chips or pretzels?**

- **Are your eating patterns similar on weekdays and weekends?**

- **Do you weigh more after a vacation?**

If You're a Clean Plate Club Eater . . .

I'm oh-so-familiar with Clean Plate Club Eaters because I am one! I love food and I love to eat. In fact, many of the strategies I recommend in this book are ones that I've used myself. Clean Plate Club Eaters do just that: they clean their plates! They'll also pick off others' plates, finish the bread basket, and eat late at night. They are fast eaters who can be triggered by snacks. They tend to be more sugar and carbohydrate sensitive. Buffets can be a disaster for CPC eaters: if it's on a plate, they'll eat it. All of it! CPCers will lose weight on vacation because they're eating three meals and not snacking. Most CPCers don't drink enough water: coffee, diet Coke, and diet Snapple are their beverages of choice. Many CPCers are veteran dieters. They've been on a host of diets and their weight has yo-yoed over the years. They often have two wardrobes—their "fat" and their "slim" clothes. They can have various food "issues" and can be emotional about eating.

How to Clean Up a Clean Plate Club Act

If you're a Clean Plate Club Eater, losing weight can be a challenge for you unless you control your environment, and that can be very difficult. The Wall Street Diet will be especially valuable for you because it covers your weakest points and helps you make decisions in advance about what to eat and how much. CPCers need to make their food life simple. They need to eliminate all but essential snacks. Eating too frequently makes

CPCers obsessed with food, while not eating often enough can make them so hungry that they make a poor food choice. If you were addicted to cigarettes or alcohol, you'd find strategies to help you avoid those substances. CPCers tend to be addicted to food. Obviously, they can't avoid food, so what they need to do is learn to embrace hunger (yes, it is OK to feel hungry for a period of time!) and to simplify their food decisions. Here are the critical considerations that will turn CPCers into success stories:

ELIMINATE DRY CARBS. Dry Carbs are refined starches such as white bread, cakes, bagels, etc. (See page 49 for details.) CPCers tend to be triggered by Dry Carbs. Just one cracker or piece of bread can send them off on a mindless eating spree. CPCers should make eliminating, or at least avoiding, Dry Carbs a high priority. My experience with clients has shown that those CPCers who work the hardest at this simple rule do the best in the long run.

DELAY JUICY CARBS TILL DINNER. Juicy Carbs are healthy whole grains and vegetables. (See page 52.) When you can manage it, it's best to enjoy your Juicy Carb at dinner time. This eliminates any possibility that even a Juicy Carb could become a trigger. Also, this tactic takes advantage of your natural ebbs and flows of willpower: most of us tend to be more in control early in the day and less in control by the end of the day. So why waste that willpower when you don't need to? Use it to keep you lean and mean during the day; relax a bit at dinner and enjoy those Juicy Carbs. They'll fill you up and keep you satisfied, and help you eliminate any late-night eating, too.

SLOW DOWN. You're moving too fast . . . You've got to make the mealtime last. For most Wall Streeters, speed is the name of the game. The faster you move, the more you achieve. While this may be true when it comes to work, it is in fact a total fat trap when it comes to eating. People who eat slowly, eat less. It takes twenty minutes for your brain to signal your stomach that you're full. If you eat your entire meal in four minutes, and then fill those remaining sixteen minutes with a few rolls from the breadbasket, some French fries from someone else's plate, and maybe a dessert order . . . Well, you can see that this approach can prompt weight gain as well as gastric distress! So relax. Put your knife and fork down at least three times in the course of the meal. Engage in conversation. Take a bathroom break. Remind yourself before each meal that you're not racing, you're not competing, you're eating. Don't rush it; enjoy it!

FOLLOW THE ¾ RULE. Make a quick judgment as soon as you're served as to what constitutes three-quarters of the meal and eat only that amount. You can push aside a quarter of the food on your plate to make it easier to hold to your decision. Or you can simply divide the plate in half. Restaurants frequently serve so much food that half a plate is quite enough.

"I've kept over thirty pounds off for five years with the Wall Street Diet. Whenever I begin to gain back a pound or two, I hear Heather's voice in my ear, reminding me about the ¾ Rule and about water and my carb picks. That gets me right back on track and into my slim pants."

—MARGARET G., CARDIOTHORACIC SURGEON

MANAGE SNACKS. Snacks are dangerous for CPCers. They can set off mindless eating that turns into way too many calories way too quickly. In fact, the reason that CPCers tend to lose weight or at least not gain while on vacation, even though they're eating high-calorie foods, is that they're not snacking all day. CPCers have to ask themselves two questions so that they can make their snack habits work for, instead of against, them.

- First: Does an afternoon snack help you eat less at dinner? If the answer is no, then you should skip an afternoon snack and stick to three meals, no snacks. If, on the other hand, you discover through trial and error that an afternoon snack helps you cut food intake at dinner, then you should make an afternoon snack part of your daily routine.

- Second: If you do qualify for an afternoon snack because it helps cut your dinner intake, then do any of my recommended Fun Snacks (page 63) tempt you to binge? If the answer is no, then you can go to the list and pick one. Stick to this one Fun Snack for a few weeks before changing. If the answer is yes, if one Laughing Cow cheese turns into six and you can't stop at one energy bar, then you need to limit yourself to either one piece of fruit or, alternatively, two Fiber Rich crackers. The Fiber Rich crackers are truly binge-proof. They're crunchy, filling, and satisfying, but they won't set you off. Stick with them and eat them only at recommended times, normally in the late afternoon, as I'll describe in The Plan.

EAT THREE REAL MEALS. Sounds odd, no? One common weight loss tactic is to skip breakfast in an effort to save calories. While I'm flexible about the timing of breakfast, I'm insistent about having breakfast, with some protein, each and every day. Your metabolism slows down while you sleep, and your breakfast is the signal your body needs to speed it up again and start burning those calories. If you skip breakfast, your body can slip into starvation mode, conserving the very calories you want to burn. If you're not hungry in the morning, you may be eating too much at dinner. When it comes to dinner, very few people would deliberately skip it, but some find that it sort of evaporates or rather morphs into a way too moveable feast. Indeed some of my clients, particularly the CPCers, occasionally indulge in what I call "The Wander." The Wander can begin with a small slice of pizza on the way home, and then maybe a stop at a food store that offers an array of free samples—maybe a cube or three or four or six cubes of cheese and a handful (no one is watching) of honey roasted nuts and then— land's sake!—who would have thought that a tiny slice of sugar-free blueberry pie could be so light and delicious? And, well, maybe you should skip dinner and just have a little something— just a bite—from the drive-through fast-food window on your way home . . . And by the time you arrive home, your pockets filled with tiny napkins and plastic forks and spoons, it's too late: you've done The Wander. Many clients tell me that they know the best spots in their area to hit on a Wander—the Whole Foods and Costcos that serve the best and most abundant samples. The Wander can set you back an astonishing number of calories and contribute almost nothing to your sense of satisfaction. The solution is to *always* plan three real meals each day. This will keep your hunger in manageable mode and your cravings under control. Think ahead to what your day will hold and what you will eat and when. You can't skip your afternoon snack because you forgot about it, realize you have nothing to eat at home for dinner, and find yourself lured into a Wander on your way home. I should be able to give you the Wall Street Pop Quiz any time, any day—"What's your next meal?"— and you should have a ready answer!

DELAY THE DINING. In general CPCers do well to delay a meal whenever possible and reasonable to do so. I know that you've always heard that a late dinner is bad for dieters, but I've found that CPCers often do better if their last meal is a late meal. It helps prevent late snacking. (Obviously, this works only if you don't snack before dinner!) It's the same with lunch and even breakfast. There's nothing wrong with a 10:30 A.M. breakfast if you're not hungry at 7 A.M. On weekends, if you wake up late, it's fine to skip breakfast altogether. Learn to work your hunger. Hold off a little bit before a meal.

EAT BEFORE YOU MEET. If you're going to a cocktail party or another uncontrolled eating environment, consider having a snack beforehand so you won't be tempted to raid the buffet. Have two Fiber Rich crackers and a 20-ounce bottle of water. Skip Laughing Cow or any cheese and just stick with the crackers and water. You just want to feel full; you don't want to trigger a snack massacre.

AVOID THE "POPPABLE, PICKABLE, DIPPABLE, UNSTOPPABLE." Poppable foods are foods with no discernible end. They include the obvious, like warehouse-sized bags of chips, large boxes of cereal, and chocolate samplers. They also include the less obvious, like hummus, olives, cherry tomatoes, and baby carrots. CPCers can be champion mindless eaters, and once they get started, it can be hard for them to call a halt. (As I've mentioned, as a CPCer myself, I used to regularly fall victim to the Poppable.) It's important for CPCers to avoid Poppable foods and prepare for situations where Poppable foods are featured (like cocktail parties). I'll give you lots of hints in the course of the book on how to achieve this.

BEWARE HUMMUS! *If I only had a nickel for every client who said, "Well, hummus is healthy, right?" Hummus is a dippable diet disaster. A 10-ounce container of hummus packs in 800 calories and 40 grams of carbs, the carb equivalent of 2.5 slices of bread. Add in one pita and you're up another 200 calories and 30 more grams of carbs. Your grand total: a whopping 1000 calories and 60 grams of carbs!*

EMBRACE FINITE FOOD. Have you ever dipped a spoon into a fresh pint of ice cream only to notice moments later that your spoon is scraping the bottom of the carton? CPCers need food boundaries. Left to forage, they run amok. Prepared frozen dinners are lifesavers for CPCers. They are finite. "Hand" fruit—a banana, an apple, a peach—something you can hold in your hand—is also great. Individual snack servings like Glenny's Soy Crisps or an energy bar can also be good snack choices. Cheese is a very individual thing. Some CPCers find that any type of cheese is a trigger and so they should avoid snacking on it. But others enjoy Babybel Light or Laughing Cow Light cheeses as satisfying, finite snacks. When you finish eating them, you're done. Likewise, most CPCers can't have a bowl of cereal, because it's just too hard to stop at one bowl. But they can add cereal to yogurt to give it some fiber and crunch. Putting cereal into yogurt magically turns it into a finite food. CPCers should avoid buying in bulk. You don't need a desk drawer full of energy bars or a pantry bursting with "single-serving" soy crisps. Buy only what you need for a limited time. The time spent running to a deli to buy a power bar in the afternoon will be good exercise for you.

BECOME A "PHASE EATER." Phase Eaters are those who eat the same thing for breakfast and/or for lunch for weeks on end. Many of my CPCers are Phase Eaters and I encourage this approach to weight loss. CPCers don't do well with variety. It's just too stimulating for them, and it encourages them to spend too much time thinking about food and what to eat. Variety is great when it comes to paint colors and shoe styles, and not so great when it comes to food. People who always have to think about what they're going to eat next can become obsessed by food, and this mind-set is counterproductive for those who are trying to lose weight. Research has shown that too many tastes and textures encourage you to overeat. Phase Eaters solve this problem by simplifying their food choices. They eat, say, yogurt and fruit or cottage cheese and two Fiber Rich crackers every morning for four or five weeks and then switch to something else. Or they might have the same chicken Caesar salad with light dressing for lunch for a month before switching to a turkey wrap with lettuce, tomato, and mustard and a green salad. So make life easy for yourself. Become a Phase Eater. Choose one or two breakfasts, one or two snacks, and one or two frozen dinners (if they work for you) and stick with them. You'll see that this simple step will make the diet exceptionally easy for you to follow and maintain. These meals become automatic and successful. And the weight comes off.

THE KITCHEN IS CLOSED! Learn to avoid kitchen reentry after you've finished your dinner. It's just too risky to expose yourself to the temptation of more food. Try to develop an evening routine that gets you away from the possibility of food and into an activity. Some clients shower right after eating dinner. Some brush their teeth. Anything that signals that eating is over for the day and the kitchen is closed can be effective. And once you eliminate those late-night, mindless snacking activities, you'll save countless calories.

SWEET STARVED? CPCers who wander into the kitchen at 11 P.M. for their sweet often find themselves still nibbling at midnight. The solution is to have dinner and then enjoy a piece of fruit. A hand fruit is the best choice of after-dinner sweet for a

Clean Plate Clubber. It's finite, delicious, satisfying, and it won't prompt a binge. When you've finished your fruit, you've finished eating for the night. Unless . . . (See below.)

CPCERS AND THE LOST DAY *Have you ever started out your day with a light, healthy breakfast, enjoyed a salad at lunch, and then joined an after-noon office birthday party in progress where you ate a slice of cake and, in the course of ten minutes, watched yourself transform from Dr. Jekyll into Mr. Hyde, eating anything in sight? By bedtime, you are so far out of bounds that it all seems hopeless. This is known as a "Lost Day" or a "Might-as-Well Day." Many CPCers are all-or-nothing types who can't forgive themselves for one poor food choice. They have a tendency to let that poor choice trigger a downward "Might-as-Well" spiral of one or two or twenty days of unhealthy eating. These folks often think in terms of "I'll start over on Monday . . ." Don't do this to yourself! If you fall off track with one food or one meal, count it as a slip and move on. Isn't it better to stop at those extra 300 calo-ries rather than continuing on to an extra 3000 calories? If you ate some cake or finished that bag of chips, just tell yourself, "This will not be a Lost Day," and get right back where you belong. See Bounce Back, pages 87–89, for more tips on how to get back on track and banish Lost Days.*

THE TURKEY SOLUTION. It's 11 P.M. You're absolutely starving. You're losing consciousness. Must . . . have . . . snack. What can CPCers eat, if they're really, truly hungry at night? Turkey! I dis-covered this trick myself as a tool to prevent my own evening munchies. Many diet programs allow certain types of low-calorie sweets after dinner. But I've found that this approach encourages night eating and reinforces positively a bad behavior pattern. The Turkey Solution is the best cure for late-night munchies. It's a posi-tive method for dealing with real hunger. Always make sure you have three or four quarter-pound bags of turkey in the fridge.* You

---

* If you really do not like turkey, you can substitute up to six hard-boiled egg whites.

can divide up the turkey yourself, but frankly my clients don't want to take the time to do this and so they stop at the supermarket or deli regularly and order a few quarter-pound bags of sliced turkey. Choose low-sodium turkey if you can; avoid any honey-roasted, smoked, or spiced turkey. Each bag of turkey will have only about 150 calories. If you're really hungry, it's satisfying. It's a good source of tryptophan, which can help you relax and sleep. If you're not really hungry and you just feel like munching, it will stop you in your tracks. Because enough turkey is enough. I've never yet had a client binge on sliced turkey. But it does the trick and stops the snack monster. Remember, the Turkey Solution is just plain turkey—not a party. You can't take the turkey, the Fiber Rich, and some mustard and create little bedtime sandwiches. The turkey is a functional snack that's designed to help manage hunger. You can have more than one bag if you like. Most clients tell me they have one bag, open the second bag and put it back. It's just turkey, after all!

DRINK WATER. Many CPCers are dehydrated. They drink lots of fluids—coffee, diet sodas, diet Snapple—but not enough water. I want you to pay attention to your water intake and consume 32 ounces by lunchtime and 64 ounces total in your day. If this is too much of a challenge at first, I advise you to start with a 20- to 24-ounce bottle by lunch and another of the same size in the afternoon. Eventually you can build up to the higher amounts. I also think it's best to limit the coffee to one or two cups a day, maximum, and try to eliminate the diet drinks and substitute water or club soda with citrus. Some clients tell me that they must have diet drinks. I advise that if diet soda is a nonnegotiable, they should try to cut down to one daily and to substitute club soda or seltzer with a splash of juice or slice of citrus. They should also be sure to consume at least half of their daily water requirements before they have their diet soda. Many wean themselves entirely off diet drinks in a short time.

If You're a Controlled Eater . . .

Controlled Eaters are just what you might think: they can control their eating, any place, any time. They can eat a handful of almonds and leave the rest, and they are capable of putting away a half-empty bag of chips. Either they were born with the ability to stop eating when full, or they've learned what satiety means. Nevertheless, they often eat the wrong things and the weight adds up. They're faced with so many eating challenges in the course of their daily lives that they've lost track of what and how to eat healthfully. They can gain weight on vacation because they're relaxed and eating more than usual. They tend to eat the same amounts and types of foods on weekends and weekdays, but those foods are high in calories and their portions are too large. The simple mistake common to Controlled Eaters is poor food choices. Many of my Controlled Eater clients used to be quite athletic, but as their jobs became more demanding, their time for exercise diminished. But their appetite didn't! These folks are sometimes eating for performance athletics but living the life of a desk jockey. But CEs tend to be good water drinkers and have good control when it comes to snacks. The very good news for Controlled Eaters is that they are usually quite successful at losing weight in a relatively short time. That's because once they learn the Wall Street strategies, they adopt them and the pounds melt away.

Strategies for Controlled Eaters

Controlled eaters are fortunate: they just need some guidelines and tips tailored to their busy lifestyle. They tend not to be emotional about eating and they usually know when to call it quits, but they need help in making food choices, particularly at restaurants and during travel. While much of this information will be detailed more fully in upcoming chapters, here are a few areas of focus that will reward Controlled Eaters with faster weight loss.

AVOID DRY CARBS—THAT IS, ALL WHITE, REFINED, PROCESSED CARBS. For most of my CE clients, overconsumption of these types of carbs has been largely responsible for their weight gain. Once you pay close attention and limit your Dry Carb intake, you'll see quick results on your scale. (See page 49 for more details.)

ENJOY YOUR SNACKS. Judicious snack choices will help you keep hunger at bay, and unlike a CPCer, you can have two snacks as well as your three meals. You can have that second snack either in the morning, or, more typically, at night. You'll see the list of frozen snacks I suggest that are good choices for a sweet at night for those who can enjoy just one. (See Evening Snacks for Controlled Eaters, page 63.) You'll see my Wall Street snack suggestions in The Plan (pages 61–63) and in the Wall Street Shopping List (pages 311–12).

STOCK UP. You can discover the healthy Wall Street Diet foods that you like and stock up on them so they're always at hand both at home and in the office. This will eliminate the decision making that can be your downfall. When the right choices are within reach, you will reach for them.

LEARN THE WALL STREET STRATEGIES. The Controlled Eater will find the forthcoming chapters on how to make good food choices while traveling, entertaining for business, and commuting invaluable. You'll learn what to eat in all of these situations and how to manage the eating challenges you encounter in your busy schedule. Once you incorporate these strategies into your daily life, you'll be surprised at how quickly you'll lose weight.

The Fine Print

Now that you've figured out your basic eating style—Clean Plate Clubber or Controlled Eater—you can look at a few other issues that will affect your personal approach to the Wall Street Diet.

Alcohol and Your Appetite

Alcohol can be an important consideration in any Wall Streeter's eating plan. I learned this quickly when clients would come in for an initial consultation and insist that they weren't about to stop having wine with dinner or a drink after work with clients or friends. Alcohol is a nonnegotiable for many people, but it can be a challenge for dieters because it's high in calories and can relax inhibitions and thus encourage poor food choices. So if you're going to drink alcohol, you need a strategy. First ask yourself these questions:

- Do you find that you lose food inhibitions after a drink or two? Does that first glass of wine lead to a second and third, and does the bread basket then empty itself onto your plate, and do you find yourself tucking into a bowl of shimmering crème brûlée and dunking a biscotti into some vin santo? This would be evidence of a lack of food inhibition! For some people, alcohol is a trigger to mindless eating. If this describes you, then you're better off either avoiding alcohol or sticking with drinks that you don't particularly enjoy so you can maintain control. (More on this in "Manage Alcohol," pages 133–37.)

- Alternatively, does alcohol have little or no effect on what you eat? Can you have a single glass of wine and then stop? Can you drink two glasses of wine at a dinner and still skip the bread, the string fries, and the dessert? This would mean that one or two drinks a day are not factors in your diet plan.

Are You a Slow Loser?

Roughly half of my clients are "slow losers" who generally lose weight at a slower pace than others. They always succeed in the end, it's just that their bodies seem primed for delayed weight loss. This characteristic has served them poorly in the past because they typically go on a diet for a week or two, see negligible results, and give up. This is unfortunate because they *will* lose the weight if they stick with their diet. In fact, many slow losers will lose only two to four pounds in the first month and then, from week four onward, will drop two to three pounds a week until they reach their goal. This initial slowness may be due to high job stress, hormone imbalance, insufficient sleep, dehydration, or simply the way their bodies work. Sometimes people who have been on many diets have trained their metabolism to go into "starvation mode" and conserve calories each time they try to limit food intake. Many diets promise an impressive weight loss in the first week or two. I won't make that type of claim because in my experience fast *initial* weight loss happens only with roughly half of my clients. I *have* had people—men in particular—lose as much as eight pounds in two weeks, but that's not common.

I know it can be hard, especially for busy, action-oriented people, to be patient. But the key to success when it comes to weight loss is simple consistency. Even if the scale doesn't reflect progress, your clothes almost always will: your waistband will be looser, and friends and colleagues will notice the difference in your appearance. You will definitely feel better, with higher energy levels. And as an encouragement, I'll mention here that I've frequently had clients ask me, following an initial meeting, "How long do I have to eat like this?" Months later, enjoying their shrinking waistlines and eating the same Wall Street foods and following the same recommendations, they complain when they travel or have their eating schedule disrupted in some way because they "miss their Wall Street Way." So, while I won't promise you'll lose ten pounds in five days, I will promise that once you begin to eat the Wall Street Way, you'll never look back.

Are You a Sundown Snacker?

Are you a night eater? Do you eat well during the day but snack in the evening? Do you find that a day of excellent food choices can be sabotaged in the hour before bedtime when you have an out-of-body omnivore experience, roaming your home, munching on leftovers, cheese chunks, crackers, and the candy miniatures left over from Halloween that you found in the back of the pantry? Nighttime snacking is usually more about habit than hunger. That's why even low-calorie snacks are a poor choice: they simply reinforce that habit of evening snacking. Late-night eating not only boosts your daily calorie intake, it can cause you to sleep poorly as your body is busy digesting all those snacks. You wake up tired and with a food hangover. Many of my clients who report a late-night snacking habit have never associated their erratic energy levels with their midnight fridge runs. If you have a sundown snack habit, whether you're a Controlled Eater or a Clean Plate Club Eater, you can rely on the Turkey Solution described above. It's also helpful to make the tempting munchies in your kitchen less accessible if you can't eliminate them altogether. I have one client who told me that when her children left for college it was easier for her to control her late-night eating because their snacks weren't in reach. Now when her children are home, she asks them not to have the snacks in the house and they're happy to oblige. Remember, too, to close the kitchen and divert your attention from food following dinner.

> *Do you count the hours until your BlackBerry finally goes dark and it's time for your fat-free ice cream, your baked veggie chips, and your sugar-free pudding pops? What could be bad, you ask, if you're eating only "light" at midnight? Well, night eating is a habit—a bad one—that needs to be controlled. Food of any kind, even those seemingly innocent foods, just reinforce your inclinations to munch mindlessly. So don't let "diet" foods hold you hostage; stick with the turkey snack trick if you're hungry at night. Eat right; sleep well; get thin.*

Do You Cook? Or Do You Order Out?

Some of my clients enjoy cooking; some keep nothing but mustard and quarter-pound bags of turkey in their fridges. If you cook, you'll want to make use of the Wall Street Shopping List (page 304). They provide some good recommended low-calorie, healthy foods. If you cook, your challenge is portion control and limiting quantities of food in the house—particularly if you're a CPCer. If you don't cook, review the frozen entrees that are listed in the Wall Street Shopping Lists and experiment until you find a few that you enjoy. Keep your freezer stocked with a good selection so you always have a healthy, low-calorie dinner on hand. Take some time to explore the supermarket delivery services in your area. Many of my clients rely on these services and they love the delivered portion-controlled meals. If you frequently rely on take-out food for dinner, be sure to check the Wall Street Cheat Sheets (pages 215–216) for suggestions on good choices from various types of restaurants. It's entirely possible these days to enjoy healthy, satisfying low-calorie meals without ever picking up anything but a phone and a fork.

DIALING FOR DINNER *Quite a number of grocery stores offer fresh low-calorie meals (as well as online or phone grocery and delivery services). You can order two or three or more meals for the week, and you'll have a healthy meal waiting at home for you. These meals are excellent examples of Finite Food and will help you with portion control as well as save you cooking and shopping time. For some people these meals are fantastic; for others they don't work because they eat out so frequently that the meals pile up in the fridge. Two examples are: Fresh Direct's Smart & Simple (http://www.freshdirect.com) and Peapod (http://www.peapod .com/). Here's a website that lists national as well as international food shopping sites including such chains as Albertson's: http://nebula.bus.msu .edu/grocerysurvey/LastMileWeb/list_of_grocers.html. One New York meal delivery service is www.nukitchenfoods.com.*

Are You a Water Drinker?

Do you drink water regularly or only when taking pain relievers? Water is a very important factor in the Wall Street Diet. It prevents constipation. Counterintuitively, it reduces bloat. And there's no question that adequate hydration can promote weight loss. I began to pay more attention to this subject when I noticed a pattern with many of my clients, particularly with CPCers, who tend to not drink enough water. These people would come to me frustrated because after a week or two of dieting the scale didn't seem to budge. We'd look at their food diary and they'd be eating the right foods and doing well in every way— except their water consumption. Once they upped their water intake, the pounds would begin to disappear. I saw this happen time and again, and now I'm a convert. If you're not a water drinker, pay special attention to this aspect of the diet. If you struggle to reach your water goal, start with a 20-ounce bottle of water before lunch and then drink one more 20-ounce bottle in the afternoon. The 20-ounce bottle is easy to finish and you can work up to the greater amount. Ultimately, you should try to get your 32 ounces of water in by lunch and your 64 total daily ounces by bedtime.

Are You a Veteran or Virgin Dieter?

Does this seem an odd question to ask? Well, I've learned that it's helpful for me to know if clients have been on countless diets or, alternatively, if they're people who've come to me because the weight has crept up over time and they're new to weight loss strategies. In my experience, the former category—people who are Veteran Dieters—must take a more stringent approach when they diet. Veteran Dieters are often Clean Plate Clubbers who have had ups and downs in their weight over the years, and they've been on various diets in an effort to control it.

If you're a Veteran Dieter, it's helpful to review your previous diets and learn from them. What was your most successful diet and why? Some Veterans can look back and recognize that a low-carb plan worked best for them; others might realize that a lower-fat plan with healthy carbs was their most successful approach. For whatever reasons, Veteran Dieters usually have to be more stringent in their adherence to a diet in order to lose weight; they should always go to the lower end of my recommendations when it comes to number of servings of any category of food. A good water intake is extremely effective for Veteran Dieters in promoting weight loss, and it's usually critically important that they strictly limit refined carbs and sugars—Dry Carbs. Veteran Dieters have an advantage in that they usually know their trigger foods and can steer clear of them.

Veteran Dieters often have to overcome the reduced hopes that come with years of unsuccessful diets. I had one client who would lose and gain the same twenty pounds each year, until she reached the age of thirty-five and gained fifty pounds . . . and kept it on! She had tried everything to lose weight—prepackaged foods, milk shakes, no-carb diets, weight loss clubs—and each time she'd embark on a new diet, her hopes were just a little lower, her resolve a little weaker. She'd start out motivated, but the minute she strayed (the wrong choice at a restaurant, a fattening muffin at Starbucks) she'd fall back into the "might-as-well" attitude that affects so many veteran dieters. That is, "I've already blown it, so I might as well have whatever I want . . . and maybe even some of that, in case I want it tomorrow!"

But the Wall Street Diet takes these "slips" into account by recognizing that successful weight loss is not about being perfect, it's about being practical. And because the diet takes into account nonnegotiables and those inevitable lapses, there's much less chance to feel you have to be flawless, or that a poor choice means you've fallen off your diet. In the words of General Patton, "A good plan today is better than a perfect plan tomorrow." And in the words of the client described earlier, "I used to feel that I had to 'be good' all the time on my diets, and I could never do that. Now, after six months on the Wall Street Diet and a weight loss of thirty-five pounds, I feel great! And that beats being good any day."

Virgin Dieters are quite different from Veterans. They often know little to nothing about diets. They may have never tried to reduce before. Most Virgin Dieters are baffled by their weight gain. They are commonly "circumstantial eaters": when they find themselves in an eating circumstance, they eat. Their problem is that their work often puts them in these situations, and they have no coping skills when it comes to the various force-feeding situations that they routinely endure. Unlike Veteran Dieters, who can tell you how many calories are in their lip gloss, Virgin Dieters tend to be clueless when it comes to the subtleties of various food choices. The advantage that Virgin Dieters enjoy is that they tend to lose weight fairly rapidly. Once they learn the appropriate strategies and the best choices, they're halfway home. Virgin Dieters are tremendously relieved when they realize the simplicity of the Wall Street Diet, because they have no intrinsic interest in dieting: they want fast results, they don't care how. The Wall Street Diet suits them to a "T."

There are other issues that come into play when your goal is weight loss. These include whether or not you entertain frequently for business, whether or not you travel regularly, and the length of your commute. These factors need special attention, and I have a chapter devoted to each.

Your Wall Street Eating ID Checklist

- **Are you a Clean Plate Club Eater?**

- **Are you a Controlled Eater?**

- **Does alcohol affect your food choices?**

- **Are you a slow loser?**

- **Are you a sundown snacker?**

- **Are you a water drinker?**

- **Do you cook?**

- **Are you a Veteran or a Virgin Dieter?**

- **Do you entertain frequently for business?**

- **Do you commute long hours to work?**

- **Do you travel a great deal?**

Now that you know your own personal eating ID, you'll be better prepared to match the Wall Street Diet techniques to your lifestyle and to be alert to those issues that will be significant to your success.

Dear Wall Street Diary

You have one more bit of work to do. I'd like you to do an abbreviated food journal—a Quick Journal. This is an excellent technique for taking your "eating pulse." It will give you a good idea of what your eating patterns are and what areas you might need to work on as you begin the Wall Street Diet. All that this Quick Journal requires is two days of recording. Keep track of everything you eat and drink for *one weekday* and *one weekend day*. Both of these days should be typical days for you. I know that your schedule may be very erratic, but if you travel, say, once a month, don't use your travel day for your Quick Journal day. On the other hand, if you travel more frequently, then it's best to do three days: a regular workday, a travel workday, and a weekend or at-home day. Likewise, and obviously, don't use a vacation day, a holiday, or any day that is very different from your normal routine. You can use a couple of sheets of paper, a little notebook, your computer, or even your BlackBerry to record (in which case you can use "memopad" or "tasks" or save it in "draft" as an e-mail to yourself). Whatever suits you and will be handy in the course of the day. Don't forget to log your beverages, including water, as well as your food intake. Don't worry too much about quantities—just guess as best you can. It's knowing the food categories—carbs, protein, veggies, fluids—that dominate your intake that will be helpful to you going forward.

One note: *please don't skip this step!* I'll tell you honestly as I tell my clients: if you're not ready to keep a Quick Journal, at least for a couple of days, you're not ready to commit to changing your eating habits and losing weight. So just do it!

Here's an example of one journal as submitted to me by a client:

Tuesday

7 A.M.	coffee with milk
9 A.M.	coffee with milk, about a cup of Kashi Fiber Rich cereal with soymilk at desk
10:30 A.M.	½ bagel at meeting; coffee with milk
12 NOON	(business lunch) 1 whole wheat roll, salmon, Caesar salad with dressing, 3 small roasted potatoes, coffee with milk, two small biscotti (they came with the check)
3 P.M.	a handful of pretzels; a diet Snapple
5 P.M.	coffee with milk, 1 small Danish left over from office meeting
8 P.M.	1 slice pizza; diet Coke

10:30 P.M.   (very hungry) 1 small bowl Kashi cereal with soymilk; some
                 goldfish; one large glass white wine

Here's an excerpt from an on-the-road client's journal:

Sunday
B.   Bloody Mary, Vegetable Omelet. Turkey Bacon.
L.   Tomato Soup [no cream], 1" square grilled cheese.

Sun. Night Mon (flight to London)
D.   Flight to London. Martini, W. Wine, Champagne, Lamb
          Tenderloin (about 4 oz.). Some Straw Potatoes. Small salad.
          Coffee.
B.   (3 AM NY) Special K, Whole Milk, Coffee. Real sugar.
          (No other option)
L.   Caesar Salad, w/dressing, parmesan cheese. Grilled sea bass.
          Afternoon Cocktails: (meeting) 2 glasses Champagne.
D.   (business meeting) One Martini, 6 Oysters, Real Dover Sole,
          sauce on the side. (Too much, but better than no control.) Two
          white wine, stilton & port. (Can't help it; I'm at the Ritz in
          London!)

Tuesday
B.   Bran Flakes, skim milk, fruit, OJ & coffee.
L.   Caesar Salad w/grilled shrimp. Too much dressing full of
          bacon. Didn't eat bacon. Killed me! Diet Coke, Double
          Espresso.
D.   Martini, 2 wine, Scallops (2), Venison tenderloin (8 oz.),
          Double espresso, skim milk. 1 small Lagavilin (single malt
          scotch). (I AM still in London. Will do better when home.)

In Part II, The Plan, you'll be able to look back at these sample di-
aries, as well as your own diary, and figure out the strengths and weaknesses they reveal.

•   •   •

I hope that reading this chapter has helped you see yourself in a new
light. You're no longer someone who "has no self-control" or someone
who's "undisciplined" about food. Gaining weight wasn't inevitable for

you: it was a perfect storm of stress and circumstances and too much of the wrong food, all largely the result of your lifestyle. But now you've analyzed your personal diet portfolio and you have some insight into your Wall Street Eating ID. Knowing who you are and how you eat gives you a powerful tool, and it will change the way you lose weight. You'll see. Your futures are up and your forecast is bullish. Now you need only take your new insights, apply them to The Plan in Part II, and move forward to meet your Wall Street goal.

PART TWO

The Plan

The Plan

Smart food choices = staying full longer = eating less = weight loss!

It's not rocket science. It's a basic plan and some simple, clever strategies that work. The Plan includes a few rules that are easy to remember and easy to live with, coupled with strategies that will get you through challenging situations that may have stymied you in the past.

The Plan + The Strategies = The Wall Street Diet

Now that you know your Eating ID, you also know your weak areas and the areas that you need to concentrate on. The next step is to look at what you should actually eat. First I'll explain The Template, which is a shorthand chart for what foods and categories make up the basics of the Wall Street Diet. Then I'll give you a weekly chart of sample Wall Street Meal Suggestions. These suggestions will give you lots of ideas for how the Wall Street Diet can work in real life. After that, you'll find a chart, "Your Personal Wall Street Choices," to fill out. This will help you focus on the foods and meals that work best for you. Then we'll take a look at some sample menus for different types of dieters: men and women, single and married people. Finally, I'll have some tips on your Food Diary and a personalized Shopping List for you to fill out. Once you read through this material, you'll have a clear and simple picture of how to eat the Wall Street way for permanent weight loss.

The Template

The Template is a snapshot of the Wall Street food categories, and it gives a complete overview of the building blocks of the diet. The Template isn't something you have to "learn"; all you have to do is take a look at it and then move on. The Template will give you the basics of the diet so you can then be flexible as various eating situations arise. You do not need to refer to this Template as you live with the Wall Street Diet. (Some people like to check it now and again; others study it once and never look back.) But it will help you understand my unique approach to food categories and weight loss.

As a trained nutritionist who's worked in hospital settings as well as private practice, I am wholly familiar with the details of nutrition science. But when I began to work with my Wall Street clients, I found I had to adapt some basic nutritional recommendations to the real world of stressed, busy people. It was obvious that I wouldn't succeed at helping them lose weight if I stuck slavishly to the conventional weight loss prescription of counting calories and eating specific prescribed foods while eliminating others. So I turned things inside out and started with the client: how did their lives dictate what they could and would eat, and then how could I weave good nutritional practices into that framework? Over time I developed a system that worked. The Template outlines that system. You'll see I've developed a unique system of food categories that is both simple and sensible. Best of all, it really works because it gives useful and flexible guidelines to what you can eat if you want to lose weight.

Let's take a look at The Template (pages 50–51), and I'll describe each category so you'll fully understand the basics of the diet. (You'll be filling in "Your Amount" later.)

"At age sixty, it's no longer about another failed diet, it's about learning to eat healthier and enjoying it. The deliverables include: simple menu choices, a shopping list, and a sixty-minute understanding of the food groups—Done, lost twenty pounds in four months and sustained it now for four more and counting."

—JOHN M. ZIMMERMAN, VP, INVESTOR RELATIONS AUTONATION, INC.

DRY CARBS. There's so much confusion about carbohydrates. No wonder, since both "good" and "bad" carbohydrates are called . . . *carbohydrates!* People who are carb-shy avoid *all* carbohydrates and thus miss out on important nutrients. And people who have become impatient with the no-carb diets of the last few years have gone back to embracing *all* carbs, thereby eating too many calories that provide little nutritional value. It can be hard to tell the difference between the two types of carbohydrates, which is why I've made a value judgment about carbs and divided them into two groups: the Dry Carbs (refined starches to be avoided) and the Juicy Carbs (to be embraced judiciously). Dry Carbs include white bread, white pasta, bagels, muffins, scones, brownies, Danish, cake, candy, pizza, and ice cream. (You have to imagine dry ice cream!)

When you eat Dry Carbs, your blood sugar spikes, your insulin kicks in, and then your blood sugar falls precipitously, making you feel tired and lethargic. There are three serious downsides to Dry Carbs: they have virtually no nutritional value; they tend to be high in calories; and, perhaps worst of all for Wall Streeters, they make you feel tired and sleepy. The average American eats roughly double the recommended daily servings of grains, and most of them are Dry Carbs. In fact, many people who come to see me are Dry Carb addicts. They eat them all day long. They might have a bagel for breakfast, a handful of pretzels and a scone later, too much bread at lunch and so on. They crave these foods constantly, and their days are a series of highs and lows. They don't even realize that these food choices are affecting the way they feel until they get them out of their systems. Then, suddenly, they feel calmer and steadier.

The Wall Street Diet Template

FOOD CATEGORY	RECOMMENDED AMOUNT	YOUR AMOUNT	THE FOODS
Dry Carbs	Zero		White bread, bagels, muffins, scones, candy, bread in the bread basket, pizza, ice cream, brownies, Danish, pasta, etc.
Juicy Carbs	4–7 allowed per week		*1 fist-sized portion of each of the following = 1 Juicy Carb*: baked/roasted white or sweet potato, all beans (black, kidney, etc.), brown rice, lentils, chickpeas, corn, winter squash, peas, marinara sauce
			Each of the following = 1 Juicy Carb: 2 slices whole wheat or rye bread, or for additional bread choices, see the Shopping List, page 304.
			1 sushi roll (6–8 pieces) = 1 Juicy Carb
			Any WSD approved frozen meal = 1 Juicy Carb
Fiber	1–3 servings per day		4–6 Fiber Rich crackers or Scandinavian bran crisps = 1 serving of fiber
			1 high-fiber whole wheat wrap = 1 serving of fiber
			½ cup oatmeal or ½ cup all bran or ¾ cup of Kashi Go Lean = 1 serving of fiber
Fruits	1–3 fruits per day		*Each of the following = 1 serving of fruit*: apple (small), apricots (2 small), ½ cup blueberries, 1 cup cantaloupe, ½ grapefruit, 2 clementines, ½ cup honeydew, 1 cup oranges, 1 cup peaches, 1 cup pineapple, 1 cup raspberries or strawberries, ½ banana, 12 cherries, 17 grapes
Vegetables	Unlimited (CPCers: no snacking on baby carrots or cherry tomatoes)		Asparagus, artichoke hearts, broccoli, cabbage, cauliflower, celery, chard, cucumbers, escarole, fennel, green beans, green onions, kale, lettuce, mushrooms, peppers, spinach, sprouts, tomatoes, zucchini, carrots, eggplant
Protein	Have protein at every meal. Choose baked, broiled, steamed, grilled, or poached.		*Each of the following = 1 serving of protein*: Breakfast options: 4–6 egg whites, 1–2 eggs (limit to 5 whole eggs per week), ½ cup cottage cheese, 2 slices turkey or Canadian bacon, 6–8 ounces low-fat yogurt, 1 packet or 1 scoop protein shake/powder, 1.5 tablespoons peanut butter

FOOD CATEGORY	RECOMMENDED AMOUNT	YOUR AMOUNT	THE FOODS
Protein (continued)			*Lunch/Dinner options (1 BlackBerry-sized portion = 3 ounces protein; shoot for 1–2 BlackBerrys at lunch/dinner)*: turkey, chicken, fish, shellfish, lamb, lean sirloin, buffalo, tofu, meat substitutes (check label for serving)
			Misc. protein choices: 8 ounces skim milk, 12 almonds, 1–2 mini Babybel Light or Laughing Cow Light cheese, 1 serving shredded light cheese for cooking, ¼-pound bag fresh sliced turkey (for CPCers)
Beverages	Drink 64 ounces of water per day. No juice, regular soda, and limit diet beverages.		Water, seltzer, herbal or green tea
Alcohol	One free drink allowed. 2nd counts as a Juicy Carb.		Light beer, wine, vodka, or scotch
Fats/Oils	Limit		Olive oil, cheese, avocado, nuts, canola oil, flaxseed oil, lite mayonnaise, salad dressing
Condiments	Choose wisely		*Pick*: mustard, balsamic vinegar, salsa, spices, lite soy sauce, seasonings
			Limit: sugary salad dressings (e.g., honey mustard, raspberry vinaigrette), ketchup, barbecue sauce, teriyaki sauce, red sauce
Fun Snack Optional	Less than 200 calories, low in fat, high in fiber. Eaten between lunch and dinner.		Lärabar, Luna bar, Kashi crunchy bar, Gnu Foods bar, 1.3-ounce bag Glenny's Soy Crisps (see Shopping List, pages 311–12, for complete list)
Lite Morning Fun Snack or Evening Snack (CE only)	Less than 80 calories. Limit after-dinner snacks to 3 times per week, to be eaten right after dinner.		*Each of the following = 1 serving*: Mid-morning options: 6–8 ounces Dannon Light & Fit yogurt or 0% Greek yogurt, 1–2 Laughing Cow w/ 1–2 Fiber Rich, 8 ounces skim milk, 12 almonds
			After-dinner options: Any nonfat/sugar-free Fudgsicle/Popsicle/fruit pop, sugar-free Jell-O, sugar-free pudding

For most people, eliminating or at least managing Dry Carbs is the single most important step they can take to lose weight. I have never yet had a client who binges on turkey or vegetables. I've never had to help someone manage their green bean and carrot intake. No. It's the quick, easy, convenient foods that we grab and overindulge in when we're stressed, exhausted, and tired—the dreaded Dry Carbs.

How many Dry Carbs can you have a day? You'll see that the chart says 0. It's especially important for Clean Plate Club Eaters, as well as Veteran Dieters, to do their best to eliminate Dry Carbs. But there are important exceptions to this guideline. As a general rule, you'll do best if you completely exclude Dry Carbs from your diet. But my Wall Street rule on Dry Carbs is that if you're in a situation where it's *rude* to avoid the Dry Carb, then go ahead and eat it. For example, if you're at a dinner party and someone has made lasagna, eat a small amount of it. If you're at an all-day meeting and there's nothing for breakfast but rolls and bagels, go ahead and eat one or a half of one. Don't agonize about it. You'll just count it in your weekly Juicy Carb count (which you'll read about next) and be done with it. So the goal is zero, but don't ever write off a day that includes a Dry Carb. Just record it and move on.

JUICY CARBS. Juicy carbs have taken a bad rap. Too many people are confused about them and don't know how to manage them. You need to have some Juicy Carbs in your diet because they provide important nutrients and they're also satisfying. Juicy Carbs include sweet potatoes, all beans (black, kidney, etc.), brown rice, lentils, chickpeas, corn, winter squash, peas, marinara sauce,* and any truly whole grain bread. Whole grain bread is a special consideration as a Juicy Carb because the rule is that you can eat this type of bread only if it's consumed as part of a sandwich, because in that instance, it's a Finite Food. Bread that's served any other way—as toast with breakfast, as part of a bread basket, etc., etc.—is not a Finite Food and therefore is to be avoided. My best advice is not to keep bread at

---

* A raw tomato is a vegetable; a cooked tomato—or any type of marinara sauce—is a Juicy Carb because cooking concentrates its sugars. In addition, many commercial tomato sauces have added sugars.

home and to eat it only in an unavoidable situation such as a breakfast meeting with no other food choices, grabbing something on the fly while running through an airport, or a similar instance. In addition to these, any sauces that are sweet or look like they've been thickened need to be counted as Juicy Carbs as they often have added sugar or cornstarch.

> A NOTE TO VEGETARIANS *If you are a vegetarian, you can use beans as your protein; you don't have to count them as a Juicy Carb.*

In general you can have four to seven Juicy Carbs a week. If you're a Clean Plate Club Eater or if you're a Veteran Dieter, you should aim for the lower number; if you're a Controlled Eater and/or a Virgin Dieter, or if you have more than thirty pounds to lose, you can have up to the higher amount. If you go over your Juicy Carbs for the day—with, say, a sandwich at a meeting and an extra drink at night—just balance it out later in the week.

> CARB COST AVERAGING *Banish carbohydrate confusion with Carb Cost Averaging. It's simple: ban Dry Carbs; cost average Juicy Carbs. That means the goal is no Dry Carbs and a Juicy Carb intake spread or averaged over the course of the week. Depending on what type of eater you are—CPC or CE—you'll have four to seven Juicy Carbs weekly.*

FIBER. Most diet plans and nutrition guidelines consider fiber an indigestible component of food rather than a separate category of food. I've found, however, that because so many people are carb-shy and thus avoid carbs entirely, and because Juicy Carbs are a good source of fiber but must be limited on a weight loss diet, it is more effective to assign fiber to its own separate category, thus insuring that you'll get a sufficient daily amount. USDA statistics tell us that while

65 percent of people *think* they get sufficient fiber in their diets, 80 percent of people do *not* get enough fiber, and that includes 75 percent of those who think they do! Many low-carb diets are too low in fiber, and many folks who try a low-carb diet find that they become constipated—and also that they dearly miss the crunch, texture, and satisfaction of fiber.

The Wall Street Diet takes a fresh approach and emphasizes fiber. Fiber is critical to your diet because it helps to keep you full longer, it helps to stabilize your blood sugar, it keeps your cholesterol down, and it's heart healthy. Moreover, when you have the irresistible urge to crunch, nothing satisfies like fiber. Counting fiber as a separate category also considerably softens the blow of limiting yourself to no more than seven Juicy Carbs a week. Most clients are initially dismayed at the thought that they can have only about one Juicy Carb a day, but when they learn what I count as fibers—and when they understand that they can have one to three fibers a day—all is forgiven.

So, yes, you can have one to three fiber choices a day. Veteran Dieters should go to the lower end and pick one or two at most. The fiber choices could be: crackers—I have three recommended types, including the ever-popular Fiber Rich crackers (four to six Fiber Rich crackers equal one fiber serving); one serving (as noted on the package) of cereals like oatmeal, All-Bran, Fiber One, Kashi Go Lean (see the Shopping List, pages 305–6, for others); or one high-fiber, whole wheat tortilla (like Trader Joe's or La Tortilla Factory or those on the Shopping List on page 306).

Cereal is an obvious great choice for breakfast, with skim milk or mixed into yogurt. If you're a Clean Plate Club Eater, you may have to be cautious with cereal. Cereal is only for breakfast; you can't rely on it for dinner. Stick with my recommended brands, and if you find yourself having more than a single portion, or bingeing on it, then it's better for you to rely on single-serving sizes (there are a host of single-serving oatmeal varieties) or else choose another breakfast. The tortilla wraps are great for lunch or for breakfast with egg white or Egg Beater omelets. The crackers can be enjoyed at breakfast with cottage cheese, crumbled into a lunchtime salad as croutons, or eaten as a satisfying afternoon snack with recommended cheeses. They can also be helpful when eaten right before dinner with a glass of water to help fill you up and control your calorie intake at dinner. You'll see some suggestions for these Fiber foods in the sample Weekly Menu Plans.

YOU CAN NEVER BE TOO THIN OR TOO FIBER RICH *I'm a CPC eater myself, and so I'm personally familiar with the binge risk that crackers can present. I experimented with many crunchy, low-calorie crackers, searching for something that I could recommend to my clients that would provide ample fiber and lots of satisfying crunch for few calories. But it was also important to be able to recommend a cracker that wasn't so tempting and so seductive that it would derail my clients' best intentions. Enter Fiber Rich crackers. Most of my clients have come to depend on Fiber Rich crackers as their snack of choice. They carry them in plastic soap boxes in their briefcases and carry-on bags, stash them in their bottom desk drawers, and keep them handy in their pantries at home. While some people joke that you can file your nails on them, I promise you, you will never be guilty of a Fiber Rich binge. If you eat them as recommended, as a snack—and always with lots of water—you'll find that they'll be your little Wall Street Diet life rafts, keeping you safe from the threat of formerly irresistible Dry Carbs. They're satisfying, crunchy, and yes, not too delicious!*

FRUIT. Fruit is an important part of your diet. It provides a host of nutrients as well as flavor and natural sweetness. The Plan allows one to three fruits a day. For most people, hand fruit—a fruit that fits in your palm—is a good choice. Hand fruits include apples, oranges, pears, peaches, plums, nectarines, or small bananas. One of any of these would equal one fruit. Clean Plate Clubbers might have to avoid the poppable, pickable fruits like grapes and cherries. If these fruits are not triggers for you to overeat, then a handful, or the amount that fits into your hand, equals a portion and they can be good choices. Remember that while fruit is good for you, too much is not good. Fruits, of course, have calories and need to be eaten in appropriate amounts. You have only so much room in your muscles to store the glycogen from these Juicy Carbs, and when you overload, no matter how healthy the food eaten, the excess begins to get converted to fat. And by the way, there's no "stockpiling" of fruits: you can't carry over fruit from one day to the next. I've had clients eat six fruits in a day because they missed their fruit on a previous day. This is not allowed!

VEGETABLES. Vegetables are unlimited. I've never known anyone who has gained weight from eating too many vegetables. There are just two caveats when it comes to veggie intake: Please remember that I define certain vegetables as Juicy Carbs and those vegetables must be limited. Corn, beans, peas, and chickpeas, according to The Plan, are Juicy Carbs and have to be limited to your appropriate weekly amount: from four to seven per week. The other consideration when it comes to vegetables is that there is no snacking on baby carrots or cherry tomatoes if you're a Clean Plate Club Eater. These two vegetables, while nutritious and generally low in calories, are too often abused because they're so pickable, poppable. It's easy to come home from work exhausted and mindlessly eat a pint of cherry tomatoes. This would be a high-sugar snack, as would a pile of baby carrots. Moreover, indulging in the pickable, poppables reinforces negative eating behaviors. The Wall Street Diet is dedicated to addressing these eating issues and so for CPCers eliminating these poppables is an important behavior control that is just as important as eliminating calories. Controlled Eaters can have one handful of cherry tomatoes or baby carrots if they can hold to that amount. If you follow that rule and recognize the Juicy Carb vegetables, you can go to town in the vegetable category!

PROTEIN. Protein is an excellent diet food. Protein keeps you satisfied: it can take about four hours to digest while carbs take only two. This means you feel fuller longer. Moreover, protein can boost your metabolism. One recent study found that people who ate 30 percent of their calories from protein preserved more lean body mass while losing weight than those who ate only 18 percent.* And the more lean body

* Leidy, H., N. Carnell, R. Mattes, and W. Campbell. "Higher protein intake preserves lean mass and satiety with weight loss in pre-obese and obese women." *Obesity.* 2007; 15:421–29.

mass, the more calories you burn, even at rest. Protein helps to stabilize your blood sugar and prevent mood swings.

Another plus for protein, particularly for Clean Plate Club Eaters: it's ordinarily binge-proof if you stick with lean protein sources like turkey, chicken, and fish. The Plan requires protein at each meal: breakfast, lunch, and dinner. This is very important. Many of my clients have in the past eaten only carbs at breakfast and sometimes the same at lunch. They find that once they include protein in each meal, they're no longer struggling with hunger and their moods and energy levels stabilize. My general guidelines on protein are:

- Choose lean protein like fish, turkey, chicken, egg whites, and lean beef.

- Choose protein that's grilled, steamed, broiled, baked, or poached. Avoid fried or breaded protein.

- Most people, certainly Clean Plate Club people, should avoid nuts except peanut or nut butter in individual serving packets (like Justin's, as listed in the Shopping List).

- In general, cheese is to be avoided. A bit of cheese as big as your thumb can have about 100 calories, and people are often tempted to eat large quantities. I wouldn't worry about some shaved cheese on a salad or the cheeses I recommend on the Shopping List (page 308) as snacks. But skip those big old bricks of aged cheddar or runny wheels of brie!

- Don't worry about protein amounts at breakfast because I'll spell it out for you in a few pages. If you're a Phase Eater, you'll measure your yogurt or cereal once and from then on know the correct amount.

- The portion size for lunch and dinner protein is a BlackBerry. That's about the size of a deck of cards and it's a reasonable amount of protein for a serving. Women should aim for one BlackBerry of protein for lunch and one at dinner; men can have up to two BlackBerrys of protein at both lunch and dinner.

BEVERAGES. Drink more water! That's the simple goal I set for almost all of my clients, some of whom are so busy and stressed that they're used to drinking nothing more than coffee and diet soda. Water works! It really does help with weight loss. In one study overweight women who increased their daily water intake by about four additional cups daily lost an additional 2.5 pounds over the course of a year.* Researchers aren't sure if that's because the water simply fills you up and helps to limit your caloric intake, or if it actually has an effect on the metabolism that promotes weight loss. Most people don't recognize that water consumption also affects the way you feel. Even mild dehydration—as little as a 1 to 2 percent loss of your body weight—can make you feel lethargic. Try to drink at least 64 ounces of water daily. I think it's important to try to drink 32 ounces before lunch. (If that's too difficult, start with a 20-ounce bottle.) Why? Because if you've accomplished that, you're well on your way to reaching your daily goal, no matter what distractions the afternoon throws your way. If you drink nothing but coffee in the morning, it's very hard to reach your goal by the end of the day. The easiest way to promote success is to simply make sure you have a liter bottle of water on your desk each morning. You can count sodium-free seltzer as part of your water goal but not sweetened seltzer. And make sure that at least half of your water consumption is flat water. Herbal tea counts, again only if it's unsweetened.

A NOTE ON SWEETENERS *Clients always ask about my recommendations on sweeteners. I think the best choice is to avoid the use of artificial sweeteners. There is controversy about their possible negative health effects, and in general, I think it's safer to stick with natural foods, and that includes small amounts of natural sugar. However, I realize that for people who are triggered to eat by natural sugar and who are also trying to lose weight, occasional use of artificial sweeteners is OK. If you do want to use artificial sweetener, I think Splenda is a good choice. Use no more than two to four packets a day. If you would prefer to use natural sugar and it's not a trigger for you, keep your sugar consumption (normally in coffee and/or tea) to one to two sugar packets daily (15 calories per packet).*

* Stookey, J. D., F. Constant, C. Gardner, B. M. Popkin. "Drinking water is associated with weight loss." Obesity Society Annual Meeting, Boston, MA, October 20–24, 2006.

Many of my clients are diet soda addicts. Diet soda has sodium, caffeine, and worst of all, artificial sweetener. Of these three ingredients, the artificial sweetener is the worst. It's been a controversial topic for years, but some research does hint at artificial sweeteners having a negative effect on weight loss efforts. One study found that diet drinks actually were associated with increased weight gain, although it was unclear if the negative effects were the result of the soda itself or some associated behavior. I've definitely noticed a pattern in diet soda drinkers who have difficulty losing weight despite a low-calorie diet. When they switch to water, they seem to respond better to a weight loss plan. For this reason, I don't count Crystal Light or artificially sweetened seltzer as contributing to your water intake. If you really want to have a diet soda, I suggest you reach your water intake goal first and then have one. (Most people find that they're not interested in a diet soda once they've consumed 64 ounces of water.) As to coffee, most of my clients rely on their morning coffee or tea. This is fine. But I would suggest that you limit it to one cup. The constant ups and downs of unlimited daily caffeine consumption can play havoc with your weight loss goals.

SIPS TO HIPS *It's easy to grab one or two of those tempting coffee drinks in the course of the day. They taste great and how much damage can a drink do, right? Well, some coffee drinks can pack nearly half a day's calories! The Starbucks Venti Double Chocolate Chip Frappuccino Blended Crème with whipped cream is a whopping 670 calories. And while that may be an extreme example, the popular Mocha Frappuccino is 310 calories and 12 grams of fat. Colas also pack a caloric wallop, especially the super-size colas. A "healthy" smoothie can clock in at 500 calories, and even fruit juice can have 100 to 150 calories per cup. In fact, it's instructive to know that today many of us get 20 to 50 percent of our calories from drinks. Sadly, research has shown that liquid calories—calories from beverages—are not satisfying and thus are not substituting for other calorie sources but are consumed in addition to them. So all those sips are going right to our hips. That's why water is the Wall Street beverage of choice.*

ALCOHOL. Alcohol is a nonnegotiable for many of my clients. Here is the general guideline I developed for those who want to drink alcohol: one drink is free; an additional drink must be counted as a carb in your weekly count. Keep in mind that by a drink, I mean a nonsweetened alcoholic drink like wine, beer, vodka, or scotch. Any mixed drink like a martini (I count it as mixed because of the calories and salt from olives), a margarita, a cosmopolitan, etc., is automatically considered a carb and never counts as a free drink. It's important for you to recognize, as described in your Wall Street Eating ID, the effect of alcohol on your eating behavior. If it's a trigger, you'll need to be scrupulous about limiting it. If not, you can simply count it as a carb. You'll find many helpful tips on how to handle alcohol in business situations in "Entertaining Wall Street Style," page 118.

FATS AND OILS. Fats and oils can play a surprisingly big role in weight loss because as you reduce your Dry Carbs and rely more on vegetables, salads become a more significant part of your diet. With salads come dressings, and some dressings are terribly high in fat and calories. Most people realize that a creamy dressing will generally be more calorie-rich than a balsamic vinegar–based dressing, but sometimes a dressing that seems "lite" may still have a lot of sugar and be higher in calories than you think. Some "lite" and low-fat dressings can have as many as 90 calories per 2-tablespoon serving, so you should always check. Also, and most important, a serving size of dressing is 2 tablespoons, and it's easy to use a lot more than that. So pay attention to dressings, limit the amount you use, and always look for light dressings. If you're at a restaurant and no light dressings are available, choose oil and vinegar and add them yourself, going lightly with the oil. Of course fats and oils don't show up only in dressings. Salads can already be surprisingly high in calories before the dressing is added. A Cobb salad, for example, can have up to 1200 calories due to the bacon, cheese, avocado, egg, etc. The general Wall Street recommendation on fat in salads is: limit it to two fats. So if you're having a Cobb salad, skip the cheese and bacon and egg yolk and keep the avocado and dressing. You don't want to make it tasteless; you just want to make it healthier. Of course fried foods and cream sauces and other obvious sources of fats and oils are to be avoided entirely.

> The easiest, tastiest, and healthiest dressing to make at home is just a combination of balsamic vinegar, Dijon mustard (made with white wine), and a splash of olive oil. Shake it in a jar and drizzle it on your salad. You can even add a bit of water to make it lighter and lower in calories.

CONDIMENTS. It's tempting to think that condiments don't count. How much damage can a little dab of flavor do? Well, just a tablespoon of mayonnaise has 100 calories and 10 grams of fat. Many sandwiches can include as much as two tablespoons of mayo (200 calories, 20 grams of fat), and that can add up to just about as many calories as you'd get in half a McDonald's quarter pounder (410 calories). And some sandwiches or deli salads can be loaded with mayo. That's why I've made condiments a food category: they require some attention. I've divided condiments into "pick" and "limit" (see page 51). The "pick" condiments are really unlimited, within reason. A nice slather of mustard on a turkey sandwich is fine, as is a good splash of balsamic vinegar on a salad. But when it comes to barbecue sauce, sugary salad dressings, and teriyaki sauces, you should limit your intake, as they are relatively high in calories and they also affect your blood sugar in negative ways. You can enjoy these "limit" condiments, but you have to manage them. I've found that the simplest way to do this is to count them as a Juicy Carb in your weekly tally. So that chicken teriyaki, for example, counts as one carb. If you use a little smidge of ketchup on a burger, you don't need to count it. But if you use a quarter cup, then it counts as a carb.

FUN SNACKS. A Fun Snack is an optional afternoon snack that is eaten between lunch and dinner. I came up with the term "Fun Snack" because so many clients wanted to classify the snack. "Is it a fiber?" "A protein?" I don't want people to become obsessed with categorizing foods. I want the diet to be seamless. People who are "counters"—who worry too much about the details of the plan—spend too much time thinking about food, and this is counterproductive. So I eventually realized that I needed to give this afternoon snack a name, just to distinguish it from the other food categories and to discourage the "counters" from doing their thing. The point of a Fun Snack is to keep you satisfied until dinner and help you better manage what you eat at dinner. Some people need it; others don't. Try going from lunch to dinner without a snack and see how hungry you are at dinner and how well you can manage your dinner choices. Another day, have a Fun Snack in the afternoon and see how it affects your dinner. Did you find yourself better able to manage dinner if you had a snack? Were you less distracted by hunger in the afternoon if you had a snack? A Fun Snack is a tool. It can keep you from overeating at dinner, from losing control at a cocktail party, and from nibbling at an office party.

A NOTE ON SNACKS *If you never snacked before, don't start now! Unless it helps you control your food intake at dinner, no snack is a requirement.*

The basic "starter" Fun Snacks are listed in The Template on pages 50–51. The list includes four bars plus Glenny's Soy Crisps. If you enjoy one of these snacks, just choose one and go. If you'd prefer something else, I have a complete list of Fun Snacks on pages 311–12 of the Shopping List.

Fun Snacks are under 200 calories. Many Fun Snacks are in portion-controlled amounts. The bars, soy crisps, etc., are Finite Foods, which are self-limiting. Some CPCers will find that Fun Snacks like Fiber Rich crackers and mini cheeses are not finite enough for them: they'll go back for a third and fourth. If that describes you, then you should stick with the Finite prepackaged choices in the Fun Snack category.

Here are the Fun Snack Guidelines:

Clean Plate Club Eaters will have only one snack a day, if they need it: a Fun Snack between lunch and dinner. They can choose from the basic list on The Template, or, for more variety, they can pick something from the complete list in the Shopping List on pages 311–12. CPCers can also choose one of the Lite Morning Fun Snacks for their afternoon snack in place of the other Fun Snacks. These Lite snacks are lower in calories but may still satisfy you.

Controlled Eaters may find that the one afternoon Fun Snack is sufficient for them. Or they may need additional snacks. If the latter is the case, they can have a Lite Morning Fun Snack and/or an Evening Snack. The Lite Morning Fun Snacks are less than 80 calories.

Lite Morning Fun Snacks for CEs

- Apple or any hand fruit

- 6 ounces Dannon Light & Fit yogurt

- 5 ounces 0% fat Greek yogurt

- 1 Laughing Cow Light wedge and a Fiber Rich cracker

- 1 Babybel Light and a Fiber Rich cracker

- 2 plain Fiber Rich crackers

- 10–12 almonds

Evening Snacks for CEs

- Tofutti pops

- Edy's No Sugar Added Fruit Bars

- Sugar Free The Original Brand Popsicle

- Fudge bar with no added sugar (various brands)

- Stonyfield Farm's squeezer (freeze the yogurt tube)

- Dannon Light & Fit yogurt (freeze it)

"The Wall Street Diet really is surprisingly simple. It's the first diet I've tried that conforms to my lifestyle, not the other way around. I've lost ten pounds and gained a whole new perspective on food."

—DAVID EISNER, CEO AND PRESIDENT, THEMARKETS.COM, LLC

*"Working with Heather Bauer has educated, motivated, and empow-
ered me to adopt eating habits that have changed the way I look and
feel. Who could have imagined this? I lost fifteen pounds easily and
have kept it off. I have more energy and feel better physically. And
the eating plan is so easily adaptable to my routines. That means I
can go to restaurants, drink wine, travel, splurge on a fancy dessert,
eat at home as part of a family, all without buying special diet foods
or starving myself. Heather has helped me to find a healthy way of
life rather than a diet! I went to Heather Bauer because I wanted
help to eat better. It also surprised me that I actually feel better
when I eat right, and that the way I feel motivates me to make better
choices. I feel empowered because I can make healthy, tasty choices
and feel great about the way I look. Food doesn't control my life—
not even chocolate!"*

—ELLEN GLAESSNER, LAWYER AT LARGE INVESTMENT BANK

PORTION CONTROL *Portion control is a subject that can be quite
confusing. I make it simple. You only need to worry about three portion
sizes:*

- Juicy Carbs should be the size of your fist.

- Fruit should be eaten in the amount that fits into the
  palm of your hand.

- Protein—fish, turkey, chicken, egg whites, or lean beef—
  should be eaten in BlackBerry-sized amounts.

*That's it! If you follow the other Wall Street rules about snacks, the
¾ Rule when dining out, ruling out Dry Carbs, etc., you really don't need
to know anything else about portion control.*

The Wall Street Meal Suggestions

Now that you understand the basics of the Wall Street Diet—The Template—let's move on to your own personalized meal choices. This will be a simple exercise. Most of my busy clients are looking for only one or two breakfast choices, a few lunch choices, and some guidelines on restaurant choices.

Following is a chart that shows a good selection of Wall Street Meal choices. Read it over and choose the breakfasts and lunches that appeal to you. Remember, all you need is one breakfast if you're a Phase Eater. Don't clutter your mind with too many choices. Pick a few lunches. And select some frozen dinners to have on hand.

> WALL STREET DIET ENTRY LEVEL *When you begin the diet, it's most effective to plan at least three days a week where you have finite lunches and dinners (like a turkey sandwich and a frozen dinner). This will help to limit your choices and also retrain you to eat in a more controlled way.*

Wall Street Meal Suggestions

Breakfast	**CEREALS** >5g fiber: Kashi Go Lean, Heart to Heart; Good Friends; Fiber One; Oat Bran; Back to Nature Banana Nut Multibran With ½ c low-fat milk or soy milk	**COTTAGE CHEESE** ½ c Breakstone's 1% cottage cheese w/2 Fiber Rich crackers and 1 fruit	**BARS/SHAKES TO GO** Lärabar, TLC crunchy, Nature Valley, Luna Sunrise, Gnu Foods bar, Myoplex Lite or Carb Sense ready-to-drink shake
Lunch	Business Lunch: 2 appetizers (salad and shrimp cocktail, salad and raw bar), or mixed green salad, grilled fish, and veggies	Turkey sandwich on whole wheat bread w/ lettuce, tomato, and mustard	Salad w/ turkey, chicken, dry tuna, tofu, or shrimp w/ 3 non-starchy non-marinated vegetables plus balsamic vinai-grette (optional double protein and fat for non–Veteran Dieters or those w/ 30+ lbs to lose)
Fun Snack Goal less than 200 calories	**FRUIT** Any fruit that fits in your hand	**CHIPS** Glenny's Soy Crisps, 1.3-oz bag	**YOGURT** 0–2% Fage Greek yogurt, Dannon Lite & Fit yogurt/smoothies, Stonyfield Light
Dinner	**FROZEN** Amy's under 300–380 calories Plus 1 c steamed veggies or 1 pack shirataki noodles	**GENERIC CHOICE** Protein, vegetable, optional starch	**CHINESE** Egg drop or hot and sour soup, steamed moo shoo chicken w/ 1 pancake
Lite Morning Fun Snack or Evening Snack (Under 80 calories, CE only) OPTIONAL After-dinner snack allowed 3 nights per week	1–2 Laughing Cows/ 1–2 Fiber Rich crackers	6-oz Dannon Light & Fit (freeze at night)	10–12 almonds

VEGGIE LINKS/ SAUSAGES	YOGURT	EGGS	OATMEAL
2 MorningStar Veggie Links or 2 Al Fresco apple maple chicken sausages plus 2 Fiber Rich crackers, 1 fruit	0–2% Greek yogurt with ¾ c Kashi Go Lean cereal and 1 fruit	4-egg-white omelet or Egg Beaters with Laughing Cow Light cheese or veg w/ slice of toast or Fiber Rich crackers, or 2 hard-boiled eggs w/ 2 Fiber Rich crackers and 1 fruit	1 c cooked or 1 packet McCann's, Arrowhead Mills (fruit-flavored or regular) or Quaker Oatmeal (regular or weight control)
Amy's pizza pocket, feta/spinach pocket, or tofu scramble pocket	Chicken veggie soup w/ no noodles or couscous (large), or 10 veggie (medium–large), or low-fat, dairy-free bean (medium–large)	½ c low-fat tuna or chicken salad on top of mixed greens, sliced cucumber, and tomatoes, plus 2 Fiber Rich crackers or 1 La Tortilla Factory wrap	6–8 pieces of sashimi, miso soup or green salad (½ dressing), optional oshitashi
CHEESE 1 Polly-O string cheese or 2 Laughing Cow Light or 2 Babybel Light cheeses w/2 Fiber Rich crackers	BAR Luna, Kashi crunchy, Lärabar, Gnu, Pria, Kind, Balance Bar	Orville Redenbacher Smart Pop mini bag	Crispy Delites 1-oz bag, any flavor
QUICK PICKUP ¼ rotisserie chicken (no skin), salad w/ 1–2 c steamed veggies	VEGGIE NIGHT Baked white or sweet potato, 2 measured c steamed veggies	DELIVERY SERVICE Meal from delivery service that is under 400 calories	QUICK-FIX DINNER 1 low-fat breaded chicken cutlet (Perdue or Bell & Evans) w/ ½ c marinara sauce over shirataki noodles or steamed spinach
Sugar-free Jell-O or sugar-free pudding (nighttime)	17 frozen grapes or 1 c frozen berries (nighttime)	25-cal Swiss Miss Sugar-Free Hot Cocoa Mix packets or 1 T Ghirardelli Chocolate Premium Hot Cocoa w/ 4 oz skim milk (nighttime)	Edy's No Sugar Added Fruit Bars or Sugar-Free Popsicle or Tofutti pop (nighttime)

Super Easy Wall Street Recipes

Here's a small collection of my personal favorite quick and easy recipes. These are a snap to whip up in a flash, even when you're dazed from a hard day of work. They're healthy and low in calories and really take only a few more minutes than a frozen dinner. All of the ingredients mentioned here can be found in the Wall Street Shopping List at the back of the book. Enjoy!

Wall Street Blintzes

I've made these for both breakfast and dinner. Whip together 4 to 6 egg whites until a lot of air is incorporated into the eggs (about 4 minutes). Add a dash of cinnamon and a splash of vanilla extract. You can add some Splenda, too, if you like. Pour into a nonstick omelet pan and, when eggs firm up, spread 2 tablespoons of skim ricotta or whipped cottage cheese and 2 tablespoons of blueberries onto the eggs. Flip or roll up and continue cooking for a minute or so until the eggs have completely cooked through. Enjoy with another sprinkling of cinnamon and 2 Fiber Rich crackers.

Oatmeal Pancakes

Take a packet of plain instant oatmeal and mix with 4 egg whites, a sprinkle of cinnamon, 2 tablespoons of whipped cottage cheese. Pour into a skillet to create whatever size pancake pleases you and cook until bubbles form on top. Turn and cook until done.

Best Burrito

Mix about 1 cup of Egg Beaters with about one-quarter cup of salsa or Desert Pepper black bean dip, plus 2 tablespoons of shredded, low-fat cheese. Roll up in a low-carb tortilla.

Chicken Parm Lite

Take a boneless, skinless chicken breast. Dip it in flavored Egg Beaters, then dip it in a bowl of unprocessed bran (or Fiber One or All-Bran cereal that's been whirled in the processor or blender) to coat. (Or skip this step and use a Bell & Evans low-fat, breaded chicken breast.) Bake in a Pyrex or other type of dish in a preheated 425-degree oven until the chicken is cooked through. In the last 10 minutes of cooking, cover with one-half cup of marinara sauce and sprinkle with shredded, low-fat cheese. Serve over steamed spinach or shirataki noodles.

Fish in a Package

Take a nonfishy fish like sole or tilapia or orange roughy. Put it on top of a piece of parchment paper (or aluminum foil) that is large enough to fully wrap the fish. Top with chopped cherry tomatoes, 1 tablespoon of capers, and a sprinkling of freshly ground pepper. Close up the parchment or foil, place the package on a baking sheet, and bake in a 375-degree oven for about 20 minutes. Serve on top of steamed spinach. It can also be served with a baked sweet potato.

Super Scallops

For 2 people, use 6 large sea scallops. Wrap each scallop around its perimeter with a thin slice of prosciutto. Sprinkle with pepper. Heat a skim of olive oil in a nonstick pan and add a crushed garlic clove. Sauté the scallops in the hot pan for 2 to 3 minutes on each side, just until firm. Serve with brown rice and a green vegetable. This is so delicious!

Mustard-Crusted Steak

Marinate a filet mignon or a lean flank or sirloin steak in the following marinade: minced garlic, a tablespoon of Dijon mustard, a tablespoon of Worcestershire sauce, and freshly ground pepper. Leave in the marinade for a half hour or so. Broil the steak until done to your liking. Serve with a green veggie. Any leftover flank or sirloin steak can be thinly sliced and served on greens for a delicious lunch salad.

Your Personal Wall Street Choices

Now is the time for you to go back to The Template on pages 50–51 and fill in *your* amounts in each food category. This will make it Your Template.

And now you'll select your favorite choices for various meals. Try to look ahead to your week and see which options will best fit various situations. If you know you have business dinners or lunches coming up, plan accordingly. (See "Entertaining Wall Street Style," page 118.) If you will be traveling, look ahead to your trip and be sure to read "Wall Street Travel Itinerary," page 144, for a wealth of tips. When you begin the diet, it's best to be a Phase Eater and limit your breakfast and lunch choices (if possible). Pick one or two breakfasts, one or two lunches, and one snack and stick with them for a few weeks. The Meal Suggestions (pages 66–67) will help you choose options for each category.

My breakfast picks:_____

_____

_____

My on-the-go airport/travel breakfast picks:_____

_____

_____

My mid-morning snack pick (CE only):_____

My business entertaining lunch picks (consult local restaurant menus):

_____

_____

_____

My personal at-home lunch picks:_____

_____

_____

My in-the-office lunch picks:_____

_____

_____

My on-the-go airport/travel lunch picks:_____

_____

_____

_____

My Fun Snack pick:_____

My business entertaining dinner picks (consult local restaurant menus):

_____

_____

_____

My personal at-home dinner picks:_____

_____

_____

_____

My on-the-go airport/travel dinner picks:_____

_____

_____

_____

My right-after-dinner snack pick (CE only):_____

A Note on Frozen Dinners

All Wall Streeters should have a few frozen dinners tucked away for those nights when you need a quick, satisfying, instant meal. They're also handy for weekend lunches. In general, you should choose a frozen entrée that's under 380 calories for men and under 300 calories for women for dinner. If you're eating a very late dinner, say, after 9 P.M., I think you should choose a very low-calorie entrée. For example, Amy's makes a Mexican tamale pie that is 150 calories. I like Amy's organic dinners because I think they're particularly tasty, but any of the other choices I've listed below are great.

If you're a Controlled Eater and you find that a frozen dinner really doesn't fill you up, then add a green salad, some frozen veggies (see the Shopping List for some that can be microwaved in an instant in the package they come in), or some shirataki noodles (more on these on page 82). If you're a CPCer, stick to the frozen meal alone. Some clients are shocked that I'd recommend a frozen pasta dinner, but I find these dinners very fulfilling and they satisfy the pasta craving in a good, calorie-controlled way.

Choose any of the following Amy's meals. This line is my favorite because every ingredient is organic and they taste great!

- Low-sodium veggie lasagna, stuffed shells, mac and soy cheese, Mexican tamale pie, brown rice and veggie bowl, individual pizza

- Any of the pockets (tofu scramble pocket, feta spinach pocket)

Or try some of these:

- Lean Cuisine Spa Cuisine Line (more veggies)

- Healthy Choice

- Kashi

- Smart Ones

- Cedarlane-Dr. Sears Zone

- Celentano

- South Beach

Inspirational Menus

Some people find it highly instructive—and inspirational—to see menu plans. Now, I want to make it clear to you that I never ask anyone to follow a particular weekly plan. My clients' lives just don't work that way. But it can be very helpful to see a hypothetical Wall Street Diet menu— one that might reflect what my successful clients are eating. So here are four sample menu plans.

I've found that my clients can generally be divided into two groups: the single people (who tend to have more free time on weekends, who might eat out more during the week, and who might travel more) and the family people (who spend time with their children on weekends, running from one activity to another, and who tend to travel slightly less and eat more at home). There are two sets of plans for each group: one for women, with a calorie range of between 1200 and 1500 calories; and one for men, with a calorie range between 1750 and 2000 calories. Calorie requirements, by the way, are variable. Age, activity level, weight, medications, and previous diet history all play a role in daily calorie requirements. If you have any questions about what calorie range is appropriate for you, check with a registered dietitian or health care professional. Keep in mind also that calories in restaurant meals can vary tremendously. I've done my best to calculate restaurant dishes as accurately as possible, but it's up to you to make wise choices and order carefully when you eat out.

Sample Menu Plan for Single Woman

	MONDAY	TUESDAY	WEDNESDAY	
Breakfast	*In the Airport* Coffee w/ skim, pick up Dannon Light & Fit from Starbucks and Nature Valley granola bar from Hudson News	*In Hotel* 2 poached eggs w/ lettuce and tomato and 1 slice wheat toast	*At the Desk* 1 packet Justin's nut butter, 2 Fiber Rich crackers, ½ banana	
Lite Morning Fun Snack (CE only)	Eat yogurt and granola bar on plane	SKIP	SKIP	
Lunch	*Business Lunch* Mixed green salad (small, no croutons, fat-free dressing), Dover sole (3 oz) w/ sautéed asparagus and tomatoes (1 c, w/ 1 T olive oil)	*Lunch Meeting* Grilled chicken sandwich (3 oz chicken with lettuce, tomato, and mustard on whole wheat bread) with a side mixed green salad (no croutons and 1 T fat-free salad dressing)	*"Chopt Salad Bar"* Mixed greens (3 c lettuce), turkey (3 oz) with broccoli, 2 egg whites, tomatoes, cucumbers (1 c each) and 2 T (say "light on dressing") fat-free vinaigrette dressing	
Fun Snack	1 Luna bar (peanut butter cookie)	*Snack in Airport* Gnu bar and unsweetened tea from Starbucks	Orange	
Dinner	*Business Dinner* Tomato and red onion salad (w/ 2 T vinaigrette), 4 oz filet mignon (broiled), side of sautéed wild mushrooms (1 c mushrooms sautéed in olive oil) and steamed broccoli (1 c), mixed berries (1 c), 1 glass wine	*Meeting Friend for a Drink/Food* 1 bottle Amstel Light (sip it slowly), 1 plain burger w/ the bun, lettuce, tomato, and small mixed green salad (no croutons, fat-free dressing)	*Business Dinner* Mexican: Guacamole (2 T) with sliced jicama (no chips), 4–6 oz of chicken or shrimp fajita, no tortilla, no rice, all of the sautéed onions and peppers, and ½ c black beans, 1 vodka soda with lime	
Evening Snack (CE only)	SKIP	SKIP	SKIP	

THURSDAY	FRIDAY	SATURDAY	SUNDAY
Pick Up at Deli en Route to Office ½ cup 1% cottage cheese (eat only ½ container) plus 2 Fiber Rich crackers	*Prepared at Home and Eaten at Desk* 5 oz 0% Greek yogurt w/ ½ c Kashi Go Lean mixed in and 1 medium plum	*Out to a Late Brunch* Order a 4-egg-white omelet (made with Pam) w/ 2 oz soft goat cheese, spinach (1 c), and sliced tomatoes	Amy's Tofu Scramble Pocket (6 oz)
Optional fruit saved from breakfast	**SKIP**		**SKIP**
In Cafeteria ¼ rotisserie chicken (no skin) w/ side green salad	Subway 6-inch wheat, sliced chicken, lettuce, tomato, mustard, 1 slice cheese, and fruit on the side (1 pack of Subway apple slices)	—	3-oz can tuna packed in water, 1 T light mayo, 1 50-calorie La Tortilla wrap (add lettuce and tomato) and 1 c low-sodium tomato soup
1 Luna bar (oatmeal raisin)	3 P.M. apple Late snack before heading to cocktail party: 1 Laughing Cow and 1 Fiber Rich cracker	¼ lb turkey plus 2 Fiber Rich crackers	*Working from Home* 1 mini bag popcorn (100 cals)
Dinner Out "Date" Rugola, radicchio, endive, and Parmesan, grilled halibut (5 oz), with steamed wild greens, share side of cauliflower puree w/ Parm (½ serving made with cream), 2 glasses wine	*Cocktail Party* 3–4 napkin rule and no dinner after: 1st napkin: 1 beef satay skewer 2nd napkin: 3 vegetable steamed dumplings 3rd napkin: 3 shrimp w/ 1 T cocktail sauce 4th napkin optional: 1 piece California roll 1 glass wine	*Dinner w/ Friends French Bistro* 5 oysters on the half shell, seared organic Atlantic salmon (5 oz) w/lentils (½ c, stir-fried) and shiitake mushrooms with almonds and curry oil, share a side of broccoli rabe, 1 vodka soda w/ lime	*Order-In Sushi* 1 mixed green salad, 1 tuna avocado roll, 4 pieces sashimi (yellowtail), 1 order oshitashi
SKIP	¼ lb turkey when home		1 Dannon Light & Fit yogurt, fruit flavored (frozen)

Sample Menu Plan for Single Man

	MONDAY	TUESDAY	WEDNESDAY	
Breakfast	*In the Airport* Medium Skim Latte (Starbucks Grande) plus 1 medium apple	*In Hotel* 3 poached eggs w/ lettuce and tomato and 1 slice whole wheat toast, a side order of mixed fruit, 1 c coffee with skim milk	*At the Desk* 1 c 1% cottage cheese w/ small fruit salad and 2 Fiber Rich crackers	
Lite Morning Fun Snack (CE only)	1 Babybel Light cheese on airplane	SKIP	SKIP	
Lunch	*Business Lunch* Mixed green salad (small, no croutons, fat-free dressing), Dover sole (6 oz) w/ sautéed asparagus and tomatoes (1 c, w/ 1 T olive oil)	*Lunch Meeting* Grilled chicken sandwich (3 oz grilled chicken with lettuce, tomato, and mustard on whole wheat bread), eat 3 more oz chicken out of 2nd sandwich with a side mixed green salad (no croutons and 1 T fat-free salad dressing)	*"Chopt Salad Bar"* Mixed greens (3 c lettuce), double turkey (6 oz) with broccoli, tomatoes, cucumbers (1 c each), olives, and 2 T (say "light on dressing") fat-free vinaigrette dressing	
Fun Snack	1 Luna bar (peanut butter cookie), 1 fruit (peach)	*Snack in Airport* Zone bar and 1 unsweetened tea from Starbucks	Medium Skim Latte (Starbucks Grande), orange	
Dinner	*Business Dinner* Tomato and red onion salad (w/ 2 T vinaigrette), 8 oz filet mignon (broiled), side of sautéed wild mushrooms (1 c of mushrooms sautéed in olive oil) and steamed broccoli (1 c), 1 glass wine	*Meeting Friend for a Drink/Food* 1 bottle Amstel Light (sip it slowly), 1 plain burger w/ the bun, lettuce, tomato, and small mixed green salad (no croutons, fat-free dressing)	*Business Dinner* Mexican: Guacamole (4 T) with sliced jicama (no chips), 8–10 oz chicken or shrimp fajita, no tortilla, no rice, all of the sautéed onions and peppers, and ½ cup black beans, 1 vodka soda with lime	
Evening Snack (CE only)	SKIP	SKIP	SKIP	

THURSDAY	FRIDAY	SATURDAY	SUNDAY
Pick Up at Deli en Route to Office 4 egg whites on multigrain English muffin with 1 slice cheese	*Prepared at Home and Eaten at Desk* 7 oz 2% Greek yogurt w/ ½ cup Kashi Go Lean mixed in and 1 medium plum	*Out to a Late Brunch* Order an egg-white veggie omelet with a side mixed green salad and a fruit salad	Amy's Breakfast Burrito (6 oz)
Small fruit salad	12 almonds		String cheese
In Cafeteria ¼ rotisserie chicken (no skin) with a bowl of veggie soup (12 oz) and a side salad (no croutons, fat-free dressing)	Subway 6-inch wheat, double turkey, lettuce, tomato, mustard, 1 slice cheese, and fruit on the side (1 pack of Subway apple slices)	—	6-oz can tuna packed in water, 1 T light mayo, 80-calorie La Tortilla wrap w/ 2 T light shredded cheese (making "tuna melt"), and 1 c low-sodium tomato soup
3 P.M. 1.3-oz bag Glenny's Soy Crisps *Hungry Before Dinner* 2 Fiber Rich crackers and 2 Baby-bel Light cheeses	1 Kashi Go Lean roll bar (caramel peanut) *Late Snack Before Heading to Cocktail Party* 2 Laughing Cow Light cheeses, 2 Fiber Rich crackers	¼ lb turkey plus 2 Fiber Rich crackers, Luna bar, 1 medium fruit (apple)	*Working from Home* 1 Laughing Cow Light cheese and 2 Fiber Rich crackers, 1 c cut-up red peppers, 1 mini bag of light popcorn w/ Tabasco sauce
Dinner Out "Date" Tuna carpaccio (or tartare), grilled swordfish (8 oz) with sautéed spinach (in olive oil), share a side of cauliflower purée w/ Parm (½ a serving made with cream), 2 glasses wine	*Cocktail Party* 3–4 napkin rule and no dinner after: 1st napkin: 3 beef satay skewers 2nd napkin: 3 vegetable steamed dumplings 3rd napkin: 6 shrimps with 2 T cocktail sauce 4th napkin: 6 pieces California roll, 2 glasses wine	*Dinner w/ Friends French Bistro* 10 oysters on the half shell, seared organic Atlantic salmon (10 oz) w/ lentils (½ cup, stir-fried) and shiitake mushrooms, share a side of broccoli rabe, 2 vodka sodas w/ lime	*Order-In Sushi* 1 mixed green salad, 1 miso soup, 1 tuna avocado roll, 6–8 pieces sashimi (yellowtail), 1 order oshitashi
SKIP	¼ lb turkey when home		1 Dannon Light & Fit yogurt, fruit flavored (frozen)

Sample Menu Plan for Family Woman

	MONDAY	TUESDAY	WEDNESDAY	
Breakfast	*Pick Up at Near-by Deli en Route to Work* Light & Fit smoothie, Luna Sunrise bar	*Order in When First Arrive at Desk* 4 scrambled egg whites (made with Pam), topped with 1 slice Monterey Jack cheese and 2 Fiber Rich crackers	*On the Go* 2 hard-boiled eggs with 2 Fiber Rich crackers and a medium fruit salad	
Lite Morning Fun Snack (CE only)	SKIP	SKIP	SKIP	
Lunch	*Conference Lunch* Premade turkey sandwich (3 oz turkey with lettuce, tomato on a roll), small fruit salad	*Lunch Ordering In* 1 tuna naruto roll (sashimi wrapped in cucumber, no rice), mixed salad	*"Chopt Salad Bar"* Mixed green salad (2 c lettuce) w/ grilled chicken (1 c chopped), green beans (½ c) red peppers (1 c), cucumbers (1 c), and 2 T vinaigrette dressing (fat-free) 2 Fiber Rich crackers	
Fun Snack	1.3-oz bag Glenny's Soy Crisps	Kashi TLC bar	Gnu Foods bar, or 2 Fiber Rich crackers and 2 Laughing Cow Light cheeses	
Dinner	*Dinner w/ Family* Mixed salad, grilled beef (lean sirloin, 4 oz) served over 2 c steamed spinach, 1 fruit optional right after dinner	*Business Dinner* 1 glass wine, mixed salad, Chicken Paillard entrée over greens (4 oz chicken), share side of steamed kale, split dessert: tiramisu	*Quick Stop at Cocktail Party (before eating dinner at home)* 1 napkin of food: 1 piece sushi (spicy tuna), 1 glass wine. No leftovers: have Amy's Mexican Tamale Pie (1 optional c steamed broccoli if starving)	
Evening Snack (CE only)	SKIP	SKIP	SKIP	

THURSDAY	FRIDAY	SATURDAY	SUNDAY
In Office Cafeteria 1 c plain oatmeal (Quaker Instant, no milk) with ½ c blueberries, cinnamon, 1 T slivered almonds, optional Splenda	*At Home* 1 bowl (¾ c) Kashi Go Lean w/ ½ cup skim milk and ½ banana	1 Kashi Go Lean waffle with ½ c whipped cottage cheese (1%) plus ½ c blueberries (making pancakes for the kids)	4-egg-white-omelet (made with Pam) w/spinach, onions (1 c total), and 1 oz soy cheddar cheese, 2 Fiber Rich crackers (making eggs for family anyway)
SKIP	SKIP	SKIP	SKIP
Business Lunch Arugula salad (3 c) w/ shaved Parm (2 oz), grilled red snapper (4 oz) served with steamed asparagus (1 c)	*Pick Up and Eat at Desk* Tuna Niçoise salad w/ no potato (can add 2 Fiber Rich crackers)	*Dinner for Lunch* Chef salad (no cheese) chopped up w/ fat-free vinaigrette dressing, 1 piece plain melba toast, 1 medium fruit (apple)	*Kids Want Fast Food* McDonald's: Grilled chicken Caesar salad w/ Newman's light vinaigrette dressing (1 packet)
Luna bar	1st snack: Tall skim cappuccino (Starbucks) 2nd snack: Pre-dinner at home, have 1 Laughing Cow Light cheese spread on 2 pieces celery	*At Another Soccer Game* Pria bar *Hungry Before Dinner* 2 slices turkey and 1 Fiber Rich cracker	*Rainy Afternoon Stuck at Home* 3 P.M.: 1 bag Glenny's Soy Crisps 5:30 P.M.: 1 sliced cucumber 7 P.M.: 4 slices turkey
Dinner Ordered in the Office Shrimp Marinara (6 large shrimp, ½ c marinara sauce) and 1 c sautéed broccoli rabe	*Pizza Night w/ Family* 1 slice pizza (Pizza Hut, 12" cheese only) and mixed salad, 1 glass wine	*Dinner Out w/ Another Couple (Thai)* Steamed fish (6 oz flounder) served w/chili, garlic, and lime in a banana leaf basket, side order of Chinese broccoli (1 c steamed), 2 glasses wine	*Dinner Ordered In (Chinese)* 1 bowl hot and sour soup (12 oz), steamed chicken (8 oz) w/mixed veggies, garlic sauce on side (ask for no sugar or cornstarch in sauce or use light soy sauce instead), 1 sugar-free chocolate pudding right after dinner
2 slices turkey when you get home	SKIP	SKIP	SKIP

Sample Menu Plan for Family Man

	MONDAY	TUESDAY	WEDNESDAY	
Breakfast	*Pick Up at Nearby Deli en Route to Work* Light & Fit smoothie, Luna Sunrise bar, and ½ banana	*Order in When First Arrive at Desk* 2 scrambled eggs (made with Pam), topped with 1 slice of Monterey Jack cheese, 2 Fiber Rich crackers, 1 optional fruit (small apple)	*On the Go* 2 hard-boiled eggs with 2 Fiber Rich crackers and a medium fruit salad	
Lite Morning Fun Snack (CE only)	SKIP	SKIP	12 raw almonds at desk	
Lunch	*Conference Lunch* Premade turkey sandwich (3 oz turkey with lettuce, tomato on a roll) plus 3 oz turkey from inside of 2nd sandwich	*Lunch Ordering In* 1 salmon naruto roll (sashimi wrapped in cucumber, no rice), 1 yellow-tail naruto roll, 1 mixed salad	*"Chopt Salad Bar"* Mixed green salad (2 c lettuce) w/ double grilled chicken (2 c chopped), ¼ avocado, red peppers (1 c), cucumbers (1 c), tomatoes (1 c), and 2 T vinaigrette dressing (fat-free)	
Fun Snack	1.3-oz bag Glenny's Soy Crisps	Kashi Go Lean roll bar	Gnu Foods bar and 1 fruit (medium apple)	
Dinner	*Dinner w/ Family* Mixed salad, grilled beef (lean sirloin, 8 oz) served over 1 c steamed spinach with a baked potato in the skin (topped with 1 T butter)	*Business Dinner* 2 glasses wine, mixed salad, 6 oz baby lamb chops with sautéed spinach, ½ cup sorbet	*Quick Stop at Cocktail Party (before eating dinner at home)* 1 napkin of food, 2 pieces sushi (spicy tuna), 1 glass wine No leftovers, have Amy's Mac and Soy Cheese and 1 optional c steamed broccoli	
Evening Snack (CE Only)	Sugar-free chocolate pudding (Jell-O)	SKIP	½ grapefruit	

THURSDAY	FRIDAY	SATURDAY	SUNDAY
In Office Cafeteria 1 c plain oatmeal (Quaker Instant, no milk) w/ ½ c blueberries, cinnamon, 1 T slivered almonds, optional Splenda	*At Home* 1 bowl Kashi Go Lean w/ ½ c skim milk and ½ banana	2 Kashi Go Lean waffles w/ ½ c whipped cottage cheese (1%) plus ½ c blueberries (making pancakes for the kids)	6-egg-white omelet (made with Pam) w/spinach, onions (1 c total), and 1 oz soy cheddar cheese, 1 multigrain English muffin (making eggs for family anyway)
1 Laughing Cow Cheese (or Mini Babybel Original) with 2 Fiber Rich crackers	1 peach and 2 Fiber Rich crackers	Orange slices at kids' soccer game (1 small orange), 1 Laughing Cow Light cheese	1 hand fruit, 12 almonds
Business Lunch Arugula salad (3 c) w/ shaved Parm (2 oz), grilled red snapper (8 oz) served with sautéed asparagus	*Pick Up and Eat at Desk* Tuna Niçoise salad w/ double tuna and no potato, 2 Fiber Rich crackers optional	*Dinner for Lunch* Chef salad (no cheese) chopped up w/ fat-free vinaigrette dressing and 1 piece plain melba toast	*Kids Want Fast Food* McDonald's: Grilled chicken Caesar salad w/ Newman's light vinaigrette dressing (1 packet), medium fruit salad
1 Lärabar	1st snack: Medium skim cappuccino (Starbucks Grande) 2nd snack: Predinner at home, have 2 Laughing Cow Light cheeses spread on 2 pieces celery	*At Another Soccer Game* Kashi Go Lean roll bar *Hungry Before Dinner* 4 slices turkey	*Rainy Afternoon Stuck at Home* 3 P.M.: Glenny's Soy Crisps 5:30 P.M.: 1 c cut-up cucumber 6 P.M.: ¼ lb turkey and 12 almonds
Dinner Ordered in the Office (Family Style Italian) Caesar salad (use 1 T dressing only), shrimp marinara (8 large shrimp, ½ c marinara sauce), and sautéed broccoli rabe (2 c cooked w/ olive oil) w/ 1 small whole wheat roll	*Pizza night w/ Family* 2 slices pizza (Pizza Hut, 12" cheese only) with a mixed salad, 1 glass wine (4 oz), 1 fruit after dinner (apple)	*Dinner Out w/ Another Couple (Thai)* Steamed fish (8-oz flounder) served with chili, garlic, and lime, served in a banana leaf basket. Side order of Chinese broccoli (1 c steamed), 2 glasses wine, 2 bites of dessert (of a fudge brownie)	*Dinner Ordered In (Chinese)* 1 bowl hot and sour soup (12 oz), steamed chicken (8 oz) with mixed veggies, ½ c brown steamed rice, garlic sauce on side (ask for no sugar or cornstarch in sauce, or use light soy sauce instead)
2 slices turkey when you get home	SKIP	Medium apple at home	SKIP

USE YOUR NOODLE *Have you heard of shirataki noodles? Shirataki noodles took the dieting world by storm not long ago because they seemed like a dieter's fantasy: a low-carb, low-calorie noodle. They are made from the flour of a yamlike Asian plant. You can find them in some supermarkets as well as some natural food stores or you can buy them online:* http://www .shiratakinoodles.net/index.html. *Some people love them; others, quite the opposite. They take some special handling, as they're sold "wet," packaged in liquid. I've had success with them using this technique: I drain them, rinse them thoroughly, and then heat them in a tablespoon or two of chicken broth. The noodles take on the flavor of the broth and then can be used to accompany a frozen dinner. If you're going to use them with a marinara sauce, you can skip the chicken broth step, as the noodles will take on the flavor of the red sauce.*

Your Personal Wall Street Diary

Keeping a food diary, especially at the beginning of your diet, is very important. It helps keep you on track. It helps you look ahead to plan your meals. And it helps you find the weak points in your eating patterns, which can be especially important if you hit a plateau. When I meet clients for the first time, I gauge their serious interest in losing weight by their willingness to log their food intake: those who resist keeping track of what they eat are usually just not ready to do the work necessary to lose weight. But most Wall Streeters are used to business plans and game plans, and familiar with the effectiveness of tracking and planning. Some clients keep a meticulous food diary until they reach their goal, and then they relax. Many clients tell me that if they feel a pound or two creep back, they go right back to logging their food intake and that gets them back on track.

Dirty Deeds

My Wall Street Food Diary has a unique feature: Dirty Deeds. You'll see it down at the bottom of the page. A Dirty Deed is just what you'd think: a poor food choice. I quickly learned that if you don't leave space for Dirty Deeds, you pretend they never happened! This is human nature, of course, but it's not effective if you want to be a successful loser. You really do want to keep track of everything you eat, including that handful of M&M's from the receptionist's desk. You'll see that Dirty Deeds will help to keep you honest and will often stop you from making a poor food choice, because you know you'll have to write it down.

Goals

Another important feature of The Wall Street Food Diary are the goals. Goals are your business plan for the week. They give you something to shoot for, something to keep in the back of your mind to inspire you to stay on track. You'll see that there's a space to list your goals on the form. Most people have the same goals. Here are the primary Wall Street Weight Loss Goals:

- Eliminate Dry Carbs

- Manage Juicy Carbs

- Drink more water

- Increase fiber

- Record in your Food Diary

Choose the three goals that you think will be most important to your weight loss success and list them in your Food Diary. It really helps to write them down, as it will make you more aware of what you're trying to achieve in the week ahead.

In addition to their regular weekly food diary, many clients find it effective, especially at the beginning of the diet, to do a kind of reverse journal where they look ahead to their week and figure out their food choices in advance. Breakfast is easy because it's repetitive. Many lunches can be planned. Restaurant lunches and dinners can be anticipated by checking menu websites and making choices in advance. (See "Entertaining Wall Street Style," page 118.) Meals on the go can also be

	MONDAY	TUESDAY	WEDNESDAY	
Breakfast				
Lite Morning Fun (CE only)				
Lunch				
Fun Snack				
Dinner				
Evening Snack (CE Only)				
Exercise				
Water				
Alcohol				
Dirty Deeds				
Weekly Goals				

THURSDAY	FRIDAY	SATURDAY	SUNDAY

planned (see "The Wall Street Travel Intinerary," page 144). Advance planning can save you thousands of calories a week.

You can use any method that's convenient for you when it comes to your food diary. You can use a little dime-store notebook if you like. Or, if you're like some of my clients, you can record in the "memo" section of your BlackBerry. You can download a version that I have online at *www.WallStreetDiet.com/resources/foodsheet.pdf.* You can use your computer to log. You can copy the form that I've provided here.

Wall Street Basic Shopping

At the back of the book you'll find a complete and detailed Shopping List that will help you choose products that will promote weight loss and make losing easy. When you have finished reading the book, you'll want to refer to the list, and I know you'll find it useful and inspiring. But to speed you on your way to weight loss, I'm giving you an abbreviated list of recommended Wall Street products—a starter list. When clients come to see me for their first visit, these are the products I draw their attention to as items that are particularly useful for beginning Wall Streeters. You don't need to buy *anything* immediately: you can simply have an omelet for breakfast, a salad for lunch, and so on. (I don't want you to use the no-time-for-shopping excuse to delay beginning the diet!)

So here are the starter list products. Check the Shopping List (pages 304–15) to find specific brand-name recommendations in each category.

- Fun Snack

- Crackers

- A cereal choice (if you like cereal for breakfast)

- Yogurt (if you enjoy yogurt for breakfast)

- A frozen dinner entrée or two

- Turkey (sliced in ¼-pound bags)

Bounce Back

It's easy to start something; the challenge is sticking with it. Many of my clients, especially those who are Veteran Dieters, have experienced the "Might-as-Well" days (aka "Insert-Bad-Word-Here Day"). Perhaps you've experienced this. You start out with a great healthy breakfast, your lunch could serve as a cover shot for a weight loss magazine, and then . . . uh oh! There's a birthday party for a coworker in the late afternoon. Or you meet a friend for an after-work drink at a bar that is serving fantabulous munchies. Before you know it, you're licking whipped cream from your second slice of cake or eating your third handful of honey-roasted peanuts. Suddenly, it's a Might-as-Well day. You might as well have a slice of pizza on the way home. You might as well have a bowl of ice cream. You might as well rip open that bag of Doritos.

Might-as-Well days can be a disaster, and believe it or not, it's not the extra calories that do the damage: it's the all-or-nothing attitude that cripples your resolve. It's human nature. Many of us, especially hardworking, competitive people, feel we have to be perfect. Any slipup is viewed as a defeat. But those who are most successful over the long haul are those who have learned how to recover. This is a very important concept for dieters to consider.

Given the critical importance of managing setbacks in a diet, I long ago developed some extremely effective recovery strategies. These strategies rely on a simple concept. Each of them helps you *reset yourself.* My clients love this idea. If you have a "Might-as-Well" day, you need to do something *active*, something *concrete*, to reset your eating pattern and get you back on track. It's not enough to just say, "It's OK, I'll do better tomorrow." No! You want to do better, to take action, right now! Here's how:

A PROTEIN DAY. A Protein Day is the major reset tool used by Wall Street Dieters. It's great for the day after a major calorie overload or a Might-as-Well day. It's also terrific for the day after you've returned from a trip. It's a simple tool that gets you back into the action without delay. A Protein Day is just what it sounds like: a day in which your diet is primarily protein. It's a clean, simple meal plan that helps reset your body.

Here are the meal options for a Protein Day:

BREAKFAST: 2 eggs (any style) or a 4- to 6-egg-white vegetable omelet

LUNCH: fish, turkey, chicken, or any protein grilled over greens with vinegar (If you simply can't tolerate only vinegar, then you can use a light vinaigrette.)

SNACK: skip entirely or else choose ¼ pound turkey or a 3-ounce can of tuna (If you prefer, you can have an orange—a good source of potassium—instead.)

DINNER: same as lunch: fish, turkey, chicken, or any protein grilled over greens with vinegar (If you simply can't tolerate only vinegar, then you can use a light vinaigrette.) You can add some steamed vegetables to your dinner.

SNACK: ¼ pound sliced turkey if necessary

I normally don't recommend dairy protein choices for a Protein Day unless a client is a vegetarian or someone who can't eat eggs or meat. Dairy products tend to be more salty and so not as effective for a Protein Day as the animal proteins suggested above.

One more note on a Protein Day: clients will sometimes tell me that they can't do a Protein Day because they're not eating at home all week. This is not a valid excuse! You can actually eat every meal out and have a successful Protein Day. Breakfast can be anywhere (diner, deli), your lunch can be a chicken Ceasar with no croutons and no Parmesan and balsamic vinegar on the side. You can skip your snack if you're on the run, and at dinner you can order a mixed green salad, any grilled protein, and a steamed or sautéed veggie at any restaurant. Simple, no?

A VEGGIE NIGHT. A Veggie Night is a good reset tool after a Might-as-Well day. It's also useful on a Sunday or Monday night when you want to jump-start your week. Some clients build in a Veggie Night to their weekly menus just as a matter of routine. Veggie Nights are especially good for those times when you get home particularly late and you just want something simple and fast to satisfy you before bed. A Veggie Night is just what you'd guess: a night when your dinner is simply vegetables. The Veggie Night dinner is a baked white or sweet potato and two measured cups of steamed vegetables. The vegetables can be any vegetable of your choice from The Template. As you can microwave both the potato and the vegetables, your Veggie Dinner can be ready in under ten minutes.

A Look Back

Now that you've had a chance to learn about The Plan and the various food categories and recommendations, let's take a quick look at the Quick Food Diary you created. (See pages 84–85 for details.) You already know if you're a Clean Plate Clubber or a Controlled Eater. Take a look at some of the other things that your diary reveals about your personal eating style:

- Count the number of carbs you ate in a typical day. Most of us are too high in this category and need to pay attention to the diet recommendations to get in line.

- How about the timing of your eating? Are you a night eater? Do you snack after dinner?

- Is there evidence in your diary that snacking affects your appetite? Do you eat a smaller meal when you've had a snack or does the snack have no effect on the amount you eat later?

- What about water and other fluids? Do you drink enough water?

- Do you eat double or triple breakfasts, perhaps because you commute?

- If you drink alcohol, does it affect the amount and type of food you eat?

- Do you eat Mishmash Dinners? Do you just have a bit of this and that all evening without having a real meal?

- Are your weekends worse than your weekdays when it comes to healthy eating?

You should now have a good picture of the weak points in your diet, and as you read ahead, you'll learn strategies that will help you manage each of your critical areas.

Weigh-Ins

Of course the point of dieting is to lose weight, and you have to keep track to measure your successes. This requires nothing more than a basic bathroom scale. Regular weigh-ins are important, but at the same time they shouldn't be emotionally charged events. You simply need a number, and it's best to try and eliminate any anxiety attached to that number. Just weigh yourself and jot down the result in your Food Diary. How often should you weigh in? You need to know yourself. If daily weigh-ins are motivating for you, do it. I've found, however, that most people are better off sticking with a weekly weigh-in on a specific day. This is because routine fluid shifts and hormonal changes can cause your weight to vary considerably on a day-to-day basis and these shifts can be discouraging. Most of my clients do well with a regular, weekly, midweek weigh-in.

So that, readers, is The Plan. It's simple. You know enough right now to begin eating the Wall Street Way. But real life, and especially a stressed work life, can make following any plan a game of Whack-a-Mole as you dodge obstacles and leap over pitfalls. The next part of the book—Part III: The Challenges—will help you anticipate almost every difficulty that daily life can throw your way.

> *"When I met Heather Bauer, I had been on diets for my entire life. She taught me how to eat to live instead of live to eat. I can go to restaurants and eat 'Heather-approved' meals. She has changed my life."*
>
> —ERICA JONG, AUTHOR

PART THREE

The Challenges

The Office Politics
of Food

Most offices are virtual toxic dumps of high-calorie, unhealthy foods, as well as minefields of tempting situations that encourage us to eat like a goose working on his foie gras. The ideal office would have carrot sticks on chilled plates readily available, nonfat yogurt and delicious fresh fruit in the kitchen area, as well as meetings held on treadmills. Doughnut eaters would be required by law to take their treats to the street and eat them huddled in the doorways with the smokers. But since that isn't going to happen any time soon, you must learn to transform your office environment into one that supports your efforts to lose weight. Of course you can't expect to mold your environment totally, so you'll also need tips to help you cope with the most challenging and socially compelling reasons to overeat with your coworkers.

Celebrate!

You say it's your birthday . . . Or maybe it's Halloween, or Groundhog Day, or even Bastille Day. It doesn't take much to get everyone in the office in the mood to party. And of course celebrations mean food. Indeed, in an office, a celebration *is* food—there's not much dancing and karaoke going on in that conference room—and usually it is high-calorie, high-fat, high-sugar . . . Just a single piece of birthday cake can pack 450 calories! It wouldn't be so bad if you could just indulge on rare occasions. But office celebrations pose a double danger: For one thing, some offices party *way* too often for your good health. For another, some of us find that what might be a simple indulgence is the first step to a "Might-as-Well" day—an abandonment of all resolutions and good intentions for that day and even for the whole week. It's a slippery slope.

> Remember that if you do indulge in a treat at an office celebration, it counts as your snack and also one of your carbs.

What to do? Consider this:

You must be a social office animal. Some people ask me if it's OK to just skip office gatherings that involve food. I don't recommend this. You work with other people, and your relationships with them are important. They're your friends and colleagues and you need to be part of the social network. On the other hand, if you work in an office that parties almost every day, that's a different story. In that instance you'd be well advised to simply skip high-cal gatherings whenever possible.

> OFFICE BUDDIES *Losing can be so much easier if you have an Office Health Buddy for moral support. I had two clients at Morgan Stanley who became Office Buddies. They were at very different levels in the company hierarchy, but they worked really well together when it came to helping each other to stick to their resolutions. They encouraged each other, sometimes split entrées at lunch, e-mailed reminders and tips. They both reached their goals and each credited the help of their buddy for making a major contribution to their success. See if there's someone in your office who would enjoy teaming with you to set and reach some healthy goals.*

Most offices typically party every few weeks, and you'll need strategies to cope with these events.

Controlled Eaters can kiss the cake. That's right: you need only bring the treat to your lips and take the smallest possible nibble. You'll be participating, enjoying the company, and spreading good cheer while maintaining your waistline.

You can always take a piece of the cake or whatever treat offered and bring it back to your office. You can then toss it out (yes, it hurts to waste food, but this particular food isn't doing you any favors) or give it to some hungry coworker.

Clean Plate Club Eaters should avoid taking even the single taste of a sweet. It's just too tempting to let that bit of sweet become the first nibble in a cascade of bad choices and Might-as-Well treats that will sabotage your day and perhaps your week. You work too hard to let that happen!

Don't, whatever you do, bring the treat back to your work area. You know why! Isn't it true that once you're alone, your fear of calories seems to evaporate? If you must, take the treat and toss it on the way out of the party or on the way back to your desk.

Some more celebration strategies:

- Have a pack of sugar-free gum or breath strips in your desk for just such occasions. Grab a piece on the way to the celebration. It will help dull your taste for sweets.

- Grab a water bottle on your way to the celebration. If your hands are busy and you're sipping, you seem to be participating even if you're not eating.

- Have at your fingertips a good excuse to refrain:

  - "No, thanks."

  - "I had a big lunch."

  - "I'm just stuffed today."

  - "I have a big dinner coming up tonight."

  - "I'm not that into sweets."

  - "We're celebrating my son's birthday tonight; I'm holding off for his cake."

- Try to be the server, not the eater. Stand near the cake and pass, pass, pass. You might even find that there's not enough left for you!

- Get your Office Health Buddy to go to celebrations with you. Sometimes another pair of eyes can help to keep you on the straight and narrow.

- Have your own "party" back at your desk. Plan to enjoy a skim latte, a bar, or a piece of fruit after the office party. You'll have something to look forward to and it will be easier to maintain control.

IT'S TIME TO LET THE AIR OUT OF "SPECIAL" *The concept of "special" gets too many hardworking folks in trouble when it comes to maintaining healthy habits on the job. Countless clients have told me that when they first started working at their interesting and exciting jobs, everything was special. They were going to amazing steak houses, flying business class, staying in luxurious hotels. One client sent me a food diary filled with two days of outrageous indulgences capped by a steak dinner, a lavish cheese plate, far too much wine, and a few glasses of port. His notes mentioned "After all, I am at Le Crillon in Paris." The good news is that it wasn't a once-in-a-lifetime experience for him. The bad news is that it wasn't a once-in-a-lifetime experience for him. When you feel that you're having a "once-in-a-lifetime" experience, of course you must indulge. But as the months go by and it becomes clear that these are not "once-in-a-lifetime" experiences, you have to transform your approach. It may be lavish and it may be extravagant, but it's not special. It may be "free," but it has a price attached and that's your figure and your health.*

The Office Kitchen

Most offices have a kitchen where workers can store food, grab a cup of coffee, and perhaps microwave a quick meal. These kitchens range from closet-sized spaces with dorm-sized fridges to extravagant rooms equipped with espresso makers and every imaginable food-prep convenience. While it's wonderful to have an office kitchen when you're trying to lose weight, it can have a downside.

The biggest complaint that my clients have about their office kitchen is food-stealing. Who knows why office environments can reduce some of us to the level of preschoolers? If this is an issue at your office, my only suggestion is to store your food in opaque containers with your name on them. Sometimes not being able to see the contents deters office snitches. If you have a tempting glass bowl of chilled fruit in the fridge, that's an invitation to all comers to have a healthy snack. You may be helping your coworkers but you're probably frustrating yourself.

Another issue with the office kitchen is the same issue that people have when they work at home: food is always available! If you can walk down the hall any time of day and grab a snack, it may be difficult for you to stick to your resolutions. Remember that a certain amount of hunger is your friend. You want to feel a bit of a pinch in your belly before you eat. If you're snacking all day, you're depriving yourself of this feeling, and you're losing touch with what actual hunger feels like. Moreover, if there's tempting food in your office kitchen, you may not be limiting yourself to the healthy snacks that you bring in.

Your everyday use of the office kitchen will depend on whether you're a Controlled or a Clean Plate Club Eater. Controlled Eaters can keep a supply of healthy foods and snacks in the office kitchen or even, if their office allows, in their own office fridge. They might stock Laughing Cow Light cheese, Babybel Light cheese, baby carrot sticks, sliced turkey, etc. Some healthy cereal and nonfat milk or low-fat soy milk are other options.

Clean Plate Club Eaters often find that the office kitchen is a dangerous place. I once had a client tell me that she'd found herself standing in her office kitchen, inhaling a box of cookies that she'd found at the back of one of the shelves. She wasn't even pausing to taste them, just absorbing them as fast as she could. It may not surprise you that she'd gone to the kitchen to heat some water for tea!

Uncontrolled eaters really must avoid the office kitchen except for planned excursions for snacks. They can keep only one or two food snacks on hand—perhaps an apple and one or two Babybel or Laughing Cow cheeses and bottled water and various types of teas. Many of my clients have asked about relying on cereal as an office snack. I think it's dangerous for uncontrolled eaters to keep any cereal in the office, healthy or otherwise. It's just too tempting to tell yourself that you're only going to have one bowl, and, after all, it's healthy, etc., etc. But CPCers know that one bowl of cereal almost inevitably leads to another and another and so on . . . When you think of snacks, the operative word should be finite. You want something with a natural ending; cereal can go on to the bottom of the box.

> Many of my clients find the results of this study painfully obvious: the *International Journal of Obesity* reported that women secretaries ate roughly two extra pieces of candy a day at work if the sweets were stored in a candy dish that was clear rather than opaque. Moreover, if the dish was on their desk, they ate two extra pieces a day as opposed to how much they ate when the dish was six feet away.* Elementary, my dear dieter? Yes, it is. But it's a good reminder: keep treats and snacks out of sight, especially if you're a Clean Plate Club Eater.

A wise alternative for Clean Plate Club Eaters is to avoid the office kitchen altogether. Keep only one food snack at your desk: a piece of fruit. If you prefer something other than fruit for an afternoon snack, keep some Fiber Rich or Scandinavian Bran Crisp crackers on hand and bring in one or two Babybel Light or Laughing Cow Light cheeses each day. Another alternative is to dash down to the deli or lobby newsstand and buy a protein bar or, if you can't pick one up locally or on your way into work, bring only one bar in each morning. See page 311 for a complete list of recommended protein bars.

* Wansink, B., J.E. Painter, and Y.K. Lee "The office candy dish: proximity's influence on estimated and actual consumption." *International Journal of Obesity* (London) 30(5) (May 2006). 871–75.

The Trojan Cake or Food Gifts

One of my clients has a very well-known store in Manhattan where she sells clothing accessories. She regularly has grateful shoppers send or drop off exquisite gifts of food to thank her for special help. She told me that once she sees these gifts, she finds it almost impossible to resist them. It's not just that they're so delicious, she said with a straight face, it's also that she feels she needs to taste them in order to write an appropriate thank-you note. Well, here's some news for those of you who would eat an entire cinnamon nut loaf in an effort to write a truly effective note: step away from the bakery box! It's time to use your imagination.

Of course it's tempting to eat a food gift. It falls into the "free food" category and, after all, someone *wants* you to eat it. But that doesn't mean you should. Here's how to handle food gifts:

- Never let the sun set on a food gift. Some people ask me if they can freeze the food and take only a taste of it as a special treat now and again. The answer is no. If the treat is in your house or your office, it will become an everyday thing. A nibble on Monday, a taste on Tuesday, a chunk on Wednesday. . . . The fact that it's taking you a long time doesn't reduce the ultimate caloric damage! If you use the "put it out of my misery" excuse and just eat it all at once, you'll just feel disappointed in yourself and defeated, as well as sickish. To avoid both these miserable paths, make sure that before the end of the day you've figured out who will be the lucky "echo" recipient of your treat.

- You can't taste a food gift if you're a Clean Plate Club Eater. In that instance, you just have to get rid of it. If you're a Controlled Eater, you can take a small sample of the food, savor it, pass it along, and immediately write your thank-you note.

- Find a home for your orphan treats. Don't feel bad about giving away a gift someone wanted you to have: they wanted to express appreciation and they did! Now you can share the pleasure with an "echo" gift. Consider in advance what to do with the treat so you don't find your resolve evaporating in a cloud of bakery-scented temptation. Here are some suggestions:

- *The conference room.* If you have a room that's used for meetings, it can be a good destination for food treats.

- *The reception desk.* Some treats—cookies or candies— can go right to the front desk to be enjoyed by visitors, messengers, and passersby.

- *The mail room.* If your office has a mail or messenger room, that can be a great end point for food treats. The staff will love it and appreciate the gesture.

- *An elderly neighbor.* Most of us know people who would be thrilled by the gift of a delicious food treat. Make their day. Spend a few minutes with them and the treat will be amplified. (Calories shed in this fashion count double!)

- *A hungry coworker.* There's often someone in the office—some perplexingly thin person—who plays the role of a human Dumpster. Be grateful for them.

Ordering In, or Conquering General Tso

"Hey, anybody want Chinese?" If you work in an office and you're trying to lose weight, that question is enough to throw you into total panic. Of course you want Chinese. You're hungry. Tired. What would be nicer than a big steaming platter of General Tso's Chicken? Preferably enough to feed a small battalion. But take a deep breath and watch these numbers dance across your diet spreadsheet: the typical order of General Tso packs in roughly 1300 calories, 3200 milligrams of sodium, and 11 grams of saturated fat. That's almost enough calories for a full day and enough sodium for a week. I guess the general was oblivious to water weight.

Many of my clients work in open areas such as trading floors. Their desks are littered with take-out menus and they order in frequently. It's fast, it's convenient, it's collegial. They can save time by not having to search for and agree on a restaurant, place an order, and wait around to be served. They can order from two or three places simultaneously, pleasing everyone. And when time is money, taking twenty minutes for lunch or dinner trumps a lost hour and a half. To be sure, part of the pleasure is gathering in someone's cube or a conference room to wolf down food while sharing war stories.

If your office regularly calls out for food deliveries, your best strategy is to be prepared. The first step you must take is to research restaurants in the neighborhood that will deliver. The best way to accomplish this is to simply take an exercise walk one day and gather actual menus. Of course you can often check restaurants online, but I find that for this purpose, it's better to have the actual menus handy in your desk. Once you have the menus, go through them and highlight the Wall Street Diet choice selections. (See the Wall Street Restaurant Menu Survival Guide, page 255.) Then, instead of feeling pressured into making a bad choice, you simply grab the menu of the appropriate restaurant and holler out, "I'll have the number 31, no sauce." No one need know that the number 31 is steamed chicken with snow peas. And remember if you order with no sauce there will always be plenty of soy sauce packets lying around, so you can drizzle just a small amount on your meal, which will suddenly be a healthy, tasty, and filling treat instead of a General Tso diet massacre.

Food Police

You've lost a few pounds. You feel really good. Your clothes are getting a bit loose and you're going to invest in a new outfit this weekend to show off the new you. Suddenly your world view has changed. Instead of being one of the gang, grabbing for the Danish and jelly doughnuts at a meeting, you're sipping tea and munching on sliced apple. But the people around you haven't changed. They're still eating mountains of food and waiting a half hour for the elevator while you dash for the stairs. As one of my male clients said to me recently, "I can't believe they eat that crap. It's so bad for them. I know I used to eat it, too, but now that I know better I'm kind of horrified." My advice to him: zip it. No one wants to hear from the newly converted that the whole office is headed for a group coronary.

My male clients, who tend to be more macho and competitive than my women clients, seem to be especially vulnerable to this impulse to become food police. I gently remind clients that they've chosen to make these healthy changes in their lives. Others can make the same choices *if they wish.* But people must make their *own* choices and no one wants to feel pressured or ridiculed into change. Coworkers also will resent criticism, expressed ("You're sure you've got enough cream cheese on that bagel?") or implied (eyes rolling as your colleague grabs a second slice of pizza).

Food is supposed to be a pleasure, whether you're dieting or not. Nothing changes the tone of a business lunch quicker than that lone person ordering "a half portion of grilled fish, no butter or fat of any kind, steamed vegetables, small salad, dressing on the side, and a club soda." Even if that's what you're going to eat, you have to be subtle and graceful when you're eating with others. (I'll give you lots of Wall Street tips on how to order "covertly" when you're enjoying business meals at a restaurant, but for now it's enough to know that it's always best to keep your diet to yourself.)

So don't comment about others' eating habits, don't get Zone food delivered to the office, don't lecture on the calorie count in the average Cheesecake Factory meal, and don't become a member of the food police. While you don't want coworkers to focus on your eating habits, it's lovely when they notice the results. When one of my clients told me that a coworker approached him in the office kitchen and quietly said, "You really look fantastic. I wonder if you'd tell me how you've managed to lose weight. Whatever you're doing is working and I think I'd like to give it a try," I felt like both my client and I had achieved a major success.

Freaky Friday

If Monday is the traditional fresh start for dieters, Friday can be the beginning of the all-too-common lost weekend. Let's face it: you're exhausted, you've held it together for five days now, there's a mood of restless, irrational exuberance in the office, and you're ready to be swept up into the party atmosphere. You've had a brilliant week and need to celebrate, or you've had a lousy week and need to forget. Whatever your week held, it's all history now and you deserve a change of pace, which usually translates into too much food and maybe too much drink.

Beware Freaky Friday. If you're prepared, you'll manage it much better than if you just slide into it, hoping for the best.

Your game plan, as always, is to plan ahead. What's your office atmosphere on Friday? Do people order in pizza every week? Many offices in Manhattan have this custom. Do people head out en masse to a local watering hole when the day winds down? Do people abandon all semblance of productive work and wander about, chatting and snacking?

On Friday morning, anticipate what's ahead of you. If you know you'll probably have pizza in the afternoon, skip your morning snack (if you're a Controlled Eater; a CPCer does not get a morning snack), consider having an energy bar and a piece of fruit for lunch, and plan a lighter than normal dinner. Don't starve yourself, as you don't want to binge later in the day, but use snacks judiciously so that your calorie intake is relatively low but you're still in shape to make good food decisions. Also, be sure to avoid the trap of thinking you "earned" that extra slice of pizza because you were careful all day. Make a decision that you're going to have one slice and that's the end. If you like to go out to dinner on Friday night, then you might want to skip the pizza and be sure to have a healthy snack on hand for the afternoon. Or does Friday night mean a relaxed dinner with your family? If so, avoid any extra snacking in the afternoon, so you can really enjoy the evening meal. Most people find that when they anticipate what the evening holds, it's easier for them to rein in the day's eating. Or make sensible substitutions. Make sure you have your healthy snack on hand if needed and that you have your excuses at the ready if you're going to skip the office pizza or other treats. Keep gum handy, if you enjoy it, to chew in the afternoon to help you stick to your guns. Carry around your water bottle so you can substitute a sip for a snack. Think ahead and you'll sail through your Fridays, enjoying the festive atmosphere while avoiding the additional calories.

One of the most important reasons to have a healthy Friday is that while Monday signals the tone of *the week*, Friday can signal the tone of *the weekend*. If you have a lost Friday, you're far more likely to have a lost weekend. I've had many clients tell me that before they came to see me they'd gotten into a routine of starting a slide on Friday afternoon that ended only on Monday morning. There seemed no point in making good choices over the weekend; they'd already, they rationalized, blown it on Friday and they figured they'd get back on track on Monday. You really can't afford to do this. It just makes your goals more difficult to meet, and it affects the way you feel—your mood, your resolve, your confidence, and your energy level. You know that when you're eating healthy meals and not overeating, you have more energy—sustained energy—than when you are bingeing. And if you're snacking all day on goodies at the office, for example, you just don't feel as well when it comes time for your relaxing dinner on Friday night.

So assess the office atmosphere on Friday and plan ahead so that the end of your week can be as positive and healthy as the beginning.

Called to the Bar

Hey, want to go grab a few? An after-work drink is often one of the perks and traditions—and sometimes obligations—of the workplace. It's not, of course, about the alcohol. It's about bonding with colleagues, meeting new business contacts, solidifying alliances, and sometimes closing the deal. Sometimes it's fun; sometimes it's work. Any way you look at it, it's a diet challenge. The main dilemma of the after-work dieter/drinker is the fact that the after-work drink comes *before* dinner and occasionally turns into dinner. Managing the challenge of after-work food and drinks is not difficult once you understand some of the issues involved. Here's how to make your after-work drinks a career-boosting event rather than a diet disaster:

Do you need to go? Clients ask me if they shouldn't just skip the drinks. As with office celebrations, you have to gauge your response in relation to your office culture. If it's a three-times-a-week event, you probably should set a limit for yourself. Perhaps you can join in once a week and pick a day that's least "dangerous" for you. Early in the week is usually better because your resolve is stronger. But don't make a blanket decision to skip *all* after-work drink dates. You'll marginalize yourself and miss out on some important aspects of your office culture. One study published in the *Journal of Labor Research* even suggested that social drinkers earn more than nondrinkers.* While I would take those results with a grain of salt, one of the lead researchers, Edward Stringham, an economics professor at San Jose State University, said, "Social drinkers are networking, building relationships and adding contacts to their BlackBerrys that result in bigger paychecks." Keep in mind that no studies have yet demonstrated that consuming large piles of chicken wings positively affects paychecks.

OUT OF SIGHT, OUT OF MIND . . . UNTIL YOU STEP ON THE SCALE!
Brian Wansink, Cornell professor and author of Mindless Eating, *created a study in which people watching the Super Bowl ate 27 percent fewer chicken wings when their plates, filled with leftover chicken bones, were left in front of them. Those who had their plates removed, lacking evidence of their consumption, ultimately ate more.** If you're having snacks at a bar or a party and the nutshells or chicken bones or empty skewers are whisked away, you'll be more inclined to overeat than if they're sitting, accusingly, in front of you. The lesson: eliminate hors d'oeuvre amnesia; the fact that you have a clean plate in front of you is not proof that you haven't eaten!*

There are drink dates and drink dates . . . There really are two different types. The most common are the casual after-work ones that include a group from the office. You can handle these basically to suit yourself. As mentioned, depending on your office culture, it's usually best to join in at least occasionally so you're in the loop on the underground office news. And, because you know these people, you can be more casual and less worried about making an impression with what you order and how long you stay and even the level of the conversation. This

---

* Peters, Bethany, and Edward P. Stringham. *No Booze? You May Lose: Why Drinkers Earn More than Nondrinkers.* Reason Foundation Policy Brief 44, pages 411–21, Los Angeles, CA: Reason Foundation, 2006.
** Wansink, B., and C.R. Payne. "Counting bones: environmental cues that decrease food intake." *Perceptual & Motor Skills* 104(1) (February 2007): 273–76.

means you can be more outspoken about, for example, claiming you want only a soft drink because you're meeting your spouse or a friend for dinner, and/or avoiding the nibbles for the same reason. But the second type of after-work drink date is the more formal one. This is the "outsider" drink date where you're meeting a business contact, perhaps someone you've never met before. Sometimes, when the suggestion of a drink date with an outsider comes up, you can simply shift the meeting to a coffee or breakfast date. Many folks are happy to have a quick, efficient morning meeting that will, due to its nature and time of day, be less time-consuming than an after-work event. It's easier to control calorie consumption in the morning, and there are healthier food choices as well.

Whatever the after-work drink occasion—whether a casual impromptu gang from the office or a formal business meeting—here are some tactics that will help you enjoy the occasion without losing control of your diet:

> **TAMP DOWN YOUR HUNGER.** There's nothing so certain as death, taxes, and chicken wings at happy hour. But bar snacks are not diet food. They tend to be fatty and salty: those inevitable chicken wings (many people are surprised to learn that they are usually fried!), pretzels, pigs in blankets, etc. If you arrive at the watering hole starving, you're at a big disadvantage. Just six chicken wings (without the celery and the blue cheese dressing) can set you back 600 calories. The solution is to plan your afternoon snack so that it will be your lifeline when it comes to bar food. Have your Fiber Rich crackers and Babybel cheese or Laughing Cow Light cheese late in the afternoon, at, say, 5 P.M. Make sure you drink plenty of water along with your snack. The goal is to arrive at the gathering place feeling full and totally in control.

> **ANTICIPATE THE EVENING.** Of course you've already had your snack so you're not starving. But you are still vulnerable to the effects that alcohol can have on your decision-making ability. Once you've had two drinks, you're less able to make a good decision

about how your food consumption will play out for the rest of the evening. So before you place your drink order and before you even think about popping a handful of nuts into your mouth, make some advance calculations. There are two effective ways to handle happy hour. If you're having just a drink or two and then heading home for a family dinner or a dinner out with someone, then your best alternative is Happy Hour Lite. Happy Hour Lite is one or two hours of convivial conversation with limited food and drink intake. Remember: you're saving yourself for later. Your goal is to avoid the dreaded double dinner. If you've decided on enjoying an HHL, I think it's best to decide in advance how long you're going to stay. When the appointed time comes, you make your graceful exit and go on to the rest of your evening. Some people find nonalcoholic drinks a good choice for an HHL. If you prefer to have an alcoholic drink, a vodka and soda or a wine spritzer is a good choice. And don't forget light beers. They range in calories from 95 to 110 each, and the carbonation makes them more filling, so it's easy to stick with one drink. If you're having a mixed drink, you can always ask the bartender to "freshen" your drink with just soda—no more alcohol—or just additional ice. Bar snacks should be avoided entirely at HHL unless there are some crudités like carrot or celery sticks to nibble on. Your afternoon snack should have stiffened your resolve, and you'll find that you'll enjoy your Happy Hour Lite and then move on to the rest of your evening without the physical and psychological burden of excess calories and possibly a lost evening. Here's a top drink picks chart, and for a fuller listing of alcoholic drinks and their calories, see the Cheat Sheets, pages 217–19.

Top Alcoholic Drink Picks and Skips

PICK	CALORIES
Glass of red or white wine (4 oz)	80–85
Light beer (12 oz)	99

White wine spritzer	45
Vodka and soda (or diet tonic)	100
Scotch on the rocks	100

SKIP	CALORIES
Margarita	300
Eggnog	305
Piña colada	465

While Happy Hour Lite is the answer for when the gathering is a prelude to something else, the Happy Hour Meal is the solution for when you have no other plans for the evening, except perhaps collapsing on the sofa with Larry King. The Happy Hour Meal is an avoidance tactic: it enables you to avoid an evening of mindless munching that can culminate in the Mishmash Dinner at home and a total calorie consumption that might be just about right if you were a lumberjack. What's an excellent, readily available Happy Hour Meal? A simple hamburger. Most burgers—without fries, cheese, and other add-ons, of course—have about 400 calories. This is a perfectly reasonable number of calories for dinner. You can have a side salad with light dressing to accompany this, but often it's simpler, especially if you're standing at the bar, to simply go with the burger. The critical issue in the Happy Hour Meal is timing: it's essential to decide that you'll go with the HHM *before* you've nibbled on wings and nuts and various other tidbits, telling yourself that these little bites couldn't possibly add up to much and, after all, they'll be your evening meal. The truth is that a few platefuls of bar food can be the equivalent of a few days' worth of calories. Moreover, when you just "nibble" the night away, you never really feel the satisfaction of having eaten a "real" meal. This can set you up for late-night eating at home, which you justify—I know, I've been there!—by telling yourself that you skipped dinner. So save your evening and save your waistline and opt for a Happy Hour Meal early on. You'll arrive home lighter and in control. See details following on specific suggestions for happy hour nibbles. See the Cheat

Sheets, starting on page 215, for a selection of specific offerings at various bars and grills.

Bar Snacks Picks and Skips

This is the horror show for dieters. Take a deep breath and just one glance down at the list of "Skips" I've listed here. Yes, it's a long list. It's meant to frighten you. You can see that a couple of hours of munching bar snacks could set you way back on your weight loss goal. This is why I often suggest that clients simply make a bar visit their dinner: skip the snacks and have a burger (no fries!) and a salad and be done with it. Now you won't be able to say you didn't know.

Bar Snacks Picks and Skips	
PICK	**CALORIES**
Vegetable crudité, no dip (Calories vary depending on amount)	25–75
SKIP	**CALORIES**
5 pretzels	60
1 handful M&M's	129
4 crackers with 1 ounce cheese	140
1 handful honey-roasted peanuts	160
5 pieces California roll	180
12 candy-coated almonds	230
3 ounces (4–5 handfuls) wasabi peas	260
2 ounces (2 handfuls) Chex Mix	246
Tortilla chips (12–15 chips)	140
1 cup guacamole	367
Nachos (small order, cheese only)	350–400
4 mozzarella sticks	431

3 martinis	480
Wings (5 wings with 3 tablespoons blue cheese dressing)	500–600
8 potato chips with dip	600
6 nachos (with beans, cheese, and ground beef)	569
(with sour cream and guacamole it is 150 calories more)	719
1 cup (5–6 handfuls) mixed nuts	875

Bar Make-a-Meals

Now that you've seen the diet nightmare that is a bar snack, you can see why I suggest you simply make happy hour a mealtime. Here are some guidelines:

Wall Street Tips for Meals at Any Bar and Grill–type Restaurant

- Consider soup and salad or a burger/sandwich with no bun or bread and a house salad.

- Opt for broth-based soups (such as vegetable or chicken noodle) instead of cream-based soups.

- Ask for a side salad or side veggie instead of French fries or onion rings.

- Most bar and grill restaurants offer a basic garden salad and are willing to add grilled chicken if requested.

- Ask about salad dressing options and choose light or fat-free options. If none are available, select a vinaigrette.

- Modify sandwich options to make them healthier by omitting cheese and bacon and by selecting mustard instead of mayo.

- Avoid dishes that have the words "crunchy" or "crispy" in the name. This usually means fried. Look for "baked," "grilled," "broiled," "steamed," "poached," or "roasted" instead.

Bar and Grill Picks and Skips

PICK	CALORIES
Chicken noodle soup (bowl)	100–200
Vegetable soup (bowl)	220
House/garden salad with low-fat/fat-free dressing	150–300
Hamburger on bun (no cheese, no sides)	350–600
Hamburger patty without bun (no cheese, no sides)	200–450
Grilled chicken sandwich (no sides, no cheese) with mustard	300–450
Grilled chicken breast without bun (no sides, no cheese)	150–300

SKIP	CALORIES
Cheese fries with creamy/cheesy dressing	2070
Chicken quesadilla	1830
Classic nachos with pico de gallo and sour cream	1450
Buffalo wings with blue cheese dressing (10 wings)	1340
Mozzarella sticks with marinara sauce (9 sticks)	1210

"I love most of the people I work with and I really enjoy my days at the office, even though they can be quite stressful. What I never appreciated, however, is that I spend so many hours of my day in situations that encourage me to eat too much! I guess I always knew this was true, but I never paid much attention to it. The result was that I'd gained over eighteen pounds in the last eight years. This was especially painful since I'm only five-four and every pound showed. The Wall Street Diet taught me to recognize these office feeding frenzies for what they are and how to avoid them or manage them.

Heather also shed light on some office friendships that were really making it hard for me to lose weight. The result? I'm down ten pounds. I still have a way to go, but I know I'll get there shortly and I know for sure I'll never get back to the weight I was."

—MARIA K., HEDGE FUND MANAGER

Psychological Issues, or It's Not All in Your Head

One of the most complicated and challenging issues that you can face when you begin to lose weight is the reactions of those around you. In an office situation, this issue can become even more confusing because the people who surround you are sometimes your direct competitors and thus may have something to win or lose as a result of your weight loss success. We hope and expect that our coworkers will support our efforts at self-improvement, but this isn't always the case. Interestingly, I've found that reactions of others often follow patterns based on gender.

THE MELTING MALE. When men lose weight, people worry about them. Even when they *should* lose weight. Here's the scenario: Jack, who's just lost thirty pounds, is alone in the elevator when Tom enters and the doors close. "Jack," whispers Tom, with a concerned look, "I've been a little worried about you. Is everything OK?" Jack is startled and answers that yes, he's fine. Better than ever in fact. Weight down, cholesterol down, blood pressure down, energy up . . . Tom nods but seems unconvinced. Days go by, and after the fourth person approaches Jack and asks if he's sick or if there's something "going on at home" or if he's sure he's all right, even *he* begins to wonder what's going on. This is disconcerting to say the least. A surprising number of male clients have told me that they have scheduled doctor's appointments because officemates repeatedly asked them if they were OK and if they should maybe get themselves "checked out." I can tell you that not one of these men got anything but a glowing report from his physician. The general medical response was: keep doing whatever you're doing. Perhaps because most men like to keep their dieting efforts to themselves, especially when it comes to coworkers, and also because many men keep their private lives quite separate from their office lives, it's understandable that coworkers might jump to the wrong conclusion about weight loss. But my advice to clients who get this sort of response to their successful weight loss is simply to smile and say, "You bet I'm fine; never better! Thanks for asking!"

LADIES WHO DON'T LUNCH. It's quite another story with many women. In a competitive office situation, a woman who loses weight is demonstrating something that may make others feel uneasy: successful weight loss is a clear sign that you are setting a goal and working toward it successfully. You're focused and determined—an achiever. Many of my clients find that as they lose weight, they also feel more energetic, more confident, and more willing to step forward in competitive situations. A very common response to this scenario at the office is some level of jealousy. Many of my women clients have been surprised by such responses from coworkers, especially from colleagues who are in great shape themselves. The genuine friend might say, "Wow, you look great! Keep it up!" The competitive coworker might comment, "Gee, you're looking really skinny. Are you still dieting?" "Skinny" or "thin" in this context have negative connotations. I believe that these subtly unenthusiastic comments are motivated by a conscious or unconscious desire to bring you "back into the herd." You're losing weight. You're demonstrating self-mastery. You're different—maybe a little better . . . You're making everyone else nervous.

Unfortunately, many women tell me that these types of comments can send them into a tailspin. They promote a powerful desire to "get back with the gang" and the most obvious and immediately satisfying way to do this is to dive into a sleeve of Oreos.

The best way to deal with comments like "You're looking very thin . . ." is to say, "Thanks a lot. I've been working hard on it." Just turn any comment around with a positive, enthusiastic response. This reinforces your confidence in what you're doing and also encourages the rest of the herd to settle down a bit.

There are other common group responses to your weight loss. Here are two that are often reported by those who've found themselves slightly uncomfortable in their new role as a slim, attractive worker.

First, there's what I call the "death of a clown." In the typical office, like the typical family, everyone has an accepted role. There's the nerd, the apple-polisher, the nurturer . . . Sometimes, when people lose weight, they throw things off balance. They've suddenly changed and they're not perceived as being the person they used to be. Maybe the overweight gal or guy was everybody's pal. But now they look different. Their behavior might have changed a bit. They're not so quick to want to grab a doughnut and a coffee and join the gang when it's time to order out. Eating, after all, is a great bonding event in an office place. Or maybe the newly slim person's behavior hasn't changed a bit, but she simply looks different. A physical change can alter the way you're perceived by the people in your life. Many people find that there's something comforting about the heavy, happy coworker. Remember when Al Roker and Star Jones lost weight? People were not universally positive about their changed appearance. Successful dieters have to cope with this challenge of altered perceptions. Maybe someone who used to be a lunch buddy no longer includes you, or maybe someone who used to confide in you seems suddenly distant. These reactions may be childish, but whoever said the office is a grown-up place?

I've had any number of clients scoff at the possibility that their office status might change as their pounds melt away, only to come to me later and confess that, yes, it's a slightly different world now that they're thinner. But most people, when they are alerted to a possible changed dynamic, are reassured and manage to cope quite gracefully with the shifting landscape. The important thing is to stick to your goals and continue with your healthy weight loss. Your coworkers will grow accustomed to the new you, and you will certainly find, as heightened energy levels and increased confidence begin to pay career dividends, that your new situation is preferable to your old one.

Another reaction that's often experienced by successful dieters is the "same old, same old." OK, you've lost a great deal of weight. The response was fabulous. You couldn't walk down a hall without having someone grab you and tell you how fantastic you look. People begged you for your diet secrets. A couple of people in the office went on diets themselves, inspired by your success. But now a few months have gone by and you haven't gotten a positive comment in weeks. What's going on? Don't you look good anymore? When folks lose weight, they normally get a lot of favorable reactions from those around them. These positive responses can be very empowering and encouraging. But as you reach your goal and maintain your weight, the comments dwindle. Some people find this discouraging, as they've become accustomed to the wonderful support of their colleagues. But you must remember that over time your coworkers simply get used to the new you. You still look great; just look in the mirror!

A rule of thumb: in general, I tell clients that any time they get negative, or less-than-supportive, feedback about their weight loss from anyone, it has more to do with the other person than with them. There's nothing like someone who's successfully working toward a goal and doing well to make other people feel inadequate and conscious of their own failings. So prepare your response to any negative comments and recognize that you are on the right path. You're making a change—a positive change—and that's why others are noticing and reacting. But competitiveness and jealousy can motivate others, particularly in a competitive situation like an office. So smile, believe in yourself, and carry on!

Friends for Lite

Many clients, most commonly women clients, have reported to me that they've found that certain friendships wreak havoc on their diets. Some of these friends are office friends; some are friends from outside of work. I'd like to briefly describe these friendships here because it's helpful to recognize when the people around you are creating obstacles to your success.

ENABLING FRIENDS. These friends mean well. They're truly fond of you and enjoy your company. But they eat too much. And too much of the wrong foods. And when you're with them, so do you. It's awkward because you don't want to make an issue of their food choices: it's not really your business. (See "Food Police," pages 101–102.) But you can't afford to do doughnut marathons. Enabling friends can be handled in a straightforward manner. If you enjoy their company and want to spend time with them, simply tell them that you're dieting. Make sure that when you meet, there are some healthy food choices for you, even if you bring them along yourself. Make light of your diet or, alternatively, mention you're working hard on it and then drop the subject. In any event, if these people are really your friends, they'll respect your choices.

TRIGGER FRIENDS. These friends are more complicated. For some reason, these people have issues that affect you in such a way they drive you to food. They may be subtly competitive. They may simply have issues that have nothing to do with you. But you find that after you see them, you feel a kind of emotional hangover that makes your dieting resolutions seem silly or pointless. Many of us have a couple of Trigger Friends in our lives. We typically manage to hold it together when we're with them, but when we get home all hell breaks loose in the kitchen. If you do have such people in your life, you shouldn't ignore the effect they have on you and you shouldn't succumb to it. Sometimes just being aware of the aftershock of Trigger Friends is enough.

CUT YOUR HAIR FRIENDS. These friends may be fun, they may be clever, but they don't have your best interests at heart. Quite the contrary. I call them "Cut Your Hair" friends because they're the ones who'd tell you you'd look great with a shaved head. That giant purple hat? Fabulous! Those white shoes that look like boats? Perfect! Cut Your Hair friends are overtly competitive. They'll encourage you to eat poorly so they'll look slimmer by contrast! Cut Your Hair friends are best enjoyed in small doses, if at all.

The Wall Street Challenge

I've mentioned the buddy system when dieting and how effective it can be. Another extremely effective tactic is to encourage your whole office to take the Wall Street Challenge. It's a simple and actually fun technique to get group support for a worthy goal. Some offices simply set a time frame and reward the person with the greatest weight loss with a specific reward— often the total pool of the $10 or $20 each participant contributes. Another alternative is to have each individual set a weight loss goal of a certain number of pounds to lose in, say, ten weeks. Everyone who reaches that goal is rewarded in some way. I've found that men usually respond to this technique best. Some women don't feel comfortable being so public with their weight loss goals. But the positive aspect of this challenge for the whole office is that it usually helps to raise consciousness about food choices and healthy food availability in the office. Everyone benefits when this happens. Check my website for more information on setting up your office Wall Street Challenge, www.WallStreetDiet.com.

"Even though I jogged and worked out with a trainer, I couldn't trim down until I started the Wall Street Diet. I love to eat—a lot. I still do, but Heather's approach was perfect for my lifestyle—and helped me understand smart and healthy eating choices. For instance, I eat at my desk almost every day, so she went online and we selected items from the menus of a bunch of nearby restaurants that deliver to my office. The results were both quick and lasting. Within weeks I'd dropped ten pounds, within a few months over thirty pounds. Two years later, the weight is still off. I now get more out of my workouts—and half a dozen folks from the gym have become Heather's clients after seeing my results."

—MARK H. HARNETT, PRESIDENT, MACKENZIE PARTNERS, INC.

Entertaining Wall Street Style: The Ins and Outs of Eating Out

Business entertaining can be a serious diet challenge. Many clients have told me that it was when they began to entertain frequently in connection with their work that they began to gain weight. You can't avoid business entertaining—it's part of your job. And of course, dining out in restaurants great and small on someone else's tab can also be fun, and profitable in terms of building business relationships. After all, you're often dining in top-notch restaurants, sampling the best your city or town has to offer, and best of all, you're not paying for it! Under those conditions, restraint has to be a conscious choice. If you're trying to lose weight, an expense account is a tender trap. There are also the simple mechanics of the situation: you need to focus on the business at hand, which is business after all, while at the same time watching what you eat without calling attention to it.

Despite the challenge of business entertaining, with a little preparation, and a recognition of the obstacles that you face, you can master all the diet minefields in restaurants. You can actually turn the tables on entertaining-related weight gain by learning how to make restaurant meals an actual opportunity to boost your nutrition and your overall health. The good news is that dining out presents terrific options for healthy eating these days. Many menus, even in common chain restaurants, offer options that are diet-friendly and health-boosting. Once you know how to navigate the system—whether you're in a diner, a take-out spot in the lobby of your office building, or a five-star restaurant—you can turn a business meal into a lean and delicious pause in your day.

Let's first take a look at some of the weight loss dilemmas that restaurants present:

LARGE PORTIONS. They think you want it. You are, or your company is, paying a lot for a meal, and most restaurants feel they must present a lavish array of food on each plate. Portion sizes in restaurants have been ballooning for the past few decades; in fact, in some cases, they've nearly doubled. This means that even a "healthy" meal can contain far too many calories.

RICH FOOD. Restaurant food is ordinarily much richer than what you might prepare yourself. It has more butter, more cream, and more salt than you would consider using at home, and sometimes these ingredients are virtually "invisible." That big knob of butter that the chef smears on top of a grilled filet mignon or swordfish steak, that double dose of dressing that turns a healthy salad into a dangerous oil spill. . . . These are just a couple of the diet disasters that trip up all but the most vigilant.

OVERORDERING. Ordering too many courses, often as a result of social pressure, can derail anyone's resolution to eat light. At home you might be happy with some grilled meat and vegetables, but at an elegant restaurant, when everyone else at the table is ordering three or four courses, it can be awkward to be the odd man out.

ALCOHOL. Pre-dinner cocktails, wine with the entrée, followed by brandy or Irish coffee. . . . There are too many opportunities to indulge while entertaining for business, and alcohol poses a double whammy: it's high in (nutritionally empty) calories and it can cloud your judgment on how much food you're consuming (and also your business dealings . . . but that's another matter!).

"MAGIC FOOD." Magic food appears out of nowhere, as if by magic, to tempt you. It's the bowl of honey-roasted peanuts that suddenly materializes at your elbow at the bar while you're waiting for your table, the overflowing bread basket that arrives with the menus, the olive-pâté crostini presented by the waiter, the "free" dessert sent out by the chef. You can scour your home of "magic food," but when you're entertaining at restaurants, you can't avoid it. These "magic foods" ambush you and can scramble even your best intentions.

FIGHT FREE FOOD WITH HEALTHY CHOICES *It's true: free food is the bane of dieters, whether it's the little paper cups of warm brownie samples at Costco, the minibar at the Ritz, or the little bag of pretzels on the plane. At least in those instances you can take a deep, cleansing breath or pop some gum in your mouth and walk on by. But when it comes to business entertaining, you can't sit there and sip on your water bottle for two hours: you have to eat. Moreover, you're not facing a few pretzels or a tiny greasy chunk of no-name pizza: you're scanning a menu that might include some of the most delicious food you've ever encountered. And you're not paying for it!*

Here's the Wall Street way to think about the free food of business entertaining: it is an opportunity to boost your nutrition with healthy choices that taste fabulous. And you don't have to shop for or prepare a thing! My clients tell me that when they scan a menu with this thought in mind, it's empowering. They no longer feel that they're depriving themselves. Rather, they view their dining-out experience as a health booster.

So how do you translate a restaurant menu into a health booster? Well, for one thing, most of us don't consume nearly enough omega-3 fatty acids, a nutrient found in cold-water fish. Many of my clients tell me that they rarely cook fish, because they don't have time to shop for it after work and they don't like frozen fish. Most restaurants these days offer a good selection of fresh fish choices. Any fish choice is good, but it's best to avoid fish that are known to be high in mercury, like swordfish and

---

bluefin tuna.* But wild salmon, striped bass, and tilapia, for example, are good choices and widely available. And if you don't like their preparations, simply ask for a fresh fish of the day, broiled or grilled. And what about vegetables? Few people eat enough of the healthy phytonutrients—or nutrients from plants—we need from vegetables. Seize the opportunity all restaurants offer: order double vegetables and skip the starch. This allows you to multiply the variety of vegetables you get in your daily diet and perhaps try some that you haven't eaten in years. (One of my clients told me that she loved escarole but never ate it because she rarely felt like cooking it. Now she makes a point of looking for it on menus.) How about fresh fruit? Is your fruit intake—an excellent source of fiber—lower than it should be? A bowl of fresh berries is a delicious and healthy dessert, and almost any restaurant will be happy to serve this even if it doesn't appear on their menu. Berries not in season or unavailable? Any fresh fruit, either plain or with some yogurt, is an excellent, healthy ending to your meal.

So turn the tables on free food and seize the opportunity to eat foods, beautifully prepared, that will make you feel and look fantastic!

Wall Street Restaurant Game Plan

You enter the restaurant and are ushered to a table of three businesspeople, none of whom you've met. You want to make a good impression and you want to forward your business objectives. You're eager to start networking. You're in the midst of introductions, trying hard to remember names and titles, when the waiter hands you a menu and asks if he can bring you a drink. This is the weakest point in a business meal for a dieter. Will you follow the crowd and order a drink, even though you don't want one, because you're distracted and everyone else is ordering wine and cocktails? Will you feel pressured into ordering an appetizer because everyone else is and you don't want to sit there calling attention to yourself while the others tuck into their Frisée aux Lardons or Crispy Calamari with Yellow String Fries?

---

* For more information on the best and safest fish choices, check *www.oceansalive.org*.

Hold on! In the world of Wall Street Dieting, rushed reflex decisions are too often bad decisions. The solution to these and many other dilemmas is, as always, to be prepared! A little time spent beforehand, recognizing the hurdles you may have to jump, will save you countless calories and pounds no matter what any business entertaining situation does to thwart you. Let's look at some strategies that will transform your restaurant experience from a potential minefield into an opportunity.

Restaurant Strategies

- Minimize your appetite.

- Limit alcohol.

- Master the menu.

- Avoid overordering.

- Seize the nutrition opportunity.

- Mask your motives (calorie counting).

- Slow down!

You're going to learn how to achieve each of these objectives. My Three-Step Restaurant Action Plan will be your blueprint to successful entertaining. When you've thought about these issues in advance, you'll find it extremely easy to implement my suggestions. My clients tell me that once they absorb these pointers, they feel in control. In this respect, business lunches and dinners become "automatic." My clients no longer agonize about choices, they no longer have to "write off" an evening because of a dining blowout; they actually feel more confident and effective in reaching their business goals, and perhaps most satisfying, they find that the pounds melt away.

The Wall Street Three-Step Restaurant Action Plan

Step One: Plan Ahead

Most business entertaining is planned in advance: the date and time and often even the restaurant are chosen and logged in on your Black-Berry or appointment calendar. This gives you a significant diet advantage. If you run through my suggested Plan Ahead strategies in the morning, you'll be well prepared to balance your meals for the day and manage any dieting dilemmas posed by a restaurant. Here are your essential plan-ahead strategies for business entertaining:

SNACK STRATEGICALLY. If you know you'll be having a late dinner out that night, you can postpone your afternoon snack until later in the day. This will prevent you from being famished when you arrive at the restaurant and thus vulnerable to the delicious smells wafting from the bread basket and the siren song of those appetizers. There's nothing worse than arriving at a restaurant so hungry that all vestiges of self-control are a distant memory. Too often my clients would eat a minimal lunch or skip it altogether to "save" their calories for later, but this plan would invariably backfire when they found themselves roaring into hunger overdrive the minute they sat down at the table. A strategic pre-dinner snack, along with plenty of water, will return you to your senses and allow you to order and eat judiciously. The ideal pre-restaurant snack is a high-fiber carb along with some protein. The best are the ones that you can keep on hand like one or two Fiber Rich crackers along with some Laughing Cow Light cheese or Babybel light cheese. Eat this a half hour to an hour before you leave for the restaurant and feel your cravings melt away.

ONE OUT OF THREE. One of the most confounding dilemmas for dieters is the pressure of having to make on-the-spot decisions when it comes to food choices. Especially in business situations, you sometimes find that either distraction, self-consciousness, or a general spirit of camaraderie promotes choices that aren't in your best interests. For that reason, I tell my clients to make a critical decision before they even enter the restaurant. Choose *one* of these three possible indulgences:

- 1 extra alcoholic drink*

- 1 piece of bread from the bread basket

- A Wall Street dessert pick, which could be one of the following (I generally suggest dessert be saved for dinner and avoided at lunch because it can be a food trigger):

  - Fruit plate

  - Fruit sorbet (except for coconut, which is relatively high in calories)

  - Biscotti (1 large or 2 small)

  - Ricotta cheesecake (not the best caloric choice but lower in sugar than chocolate or other cakes)

  - Fruit and cheese plate (good choice for those who are sugar-sensitive, but relatively high in calories)

It's amazing how much easier it is to stick with these resolutions when you make them *in advance* rather than when you're caught up in the general bonhomie of the occasion. It's when you've already had one drink and the bread basket is circling the table and you know that at least half the table will order dessert that you can find yourself falling victim to confusion or high spirits and ultimately a caloric disaster. So enjoy your extra drink or piece of bread or perhaps a small dessert. It's your choice. It's freeing to know that *you're* making the decision and enjoying the treats that are important to you.

MASTER THE MENU. Those first few moments of a business meal are totally distracting. You're often meeting new people, trying to find common ground, and thinking about the business ahead. The

---

* You are always allowed one "free" non-mixed drink; a second is counted as a carb. See Manage Alcohol, pages 133–37.

meal will go so much more smoothly if you can devote your energies right from the outset to greetings and conversation rather than to studying the menu or, worse, ordering a high-calorie choice just to get the task out of the way. If you know in advance which restaurant you'll be visiting, it's easy to check out the menu ahead of time: you can either look it up online (see page 126 for some useful sites for this purpose) or call the restaurant and have them fax you a menu. You can even check to see if there are any specials on the menu that day. If you plot it all out in advance, back in the calm and quiet of your office while you're clearheaded and not famished, you'll make better menu selections. With that out of the way, you're ready to enjoy a healthy, diet-friendly meal while making the most of the business and social opportunities.

MANAGE DISAPPOINTMENT. You ordered the broiled fish and your associate ordered the grilled chicken and you lost. Sometimes your choice is a bomb and, yes, it seems silly but the disappointment can encourage you to "compensate" with a big gooey dessert or a slab of bread. But don't let a restaurant disappointment sabotage you. Here are some solutions:

- If your menu pick isn't available or the menu has changed:

    DON'T fling yourself into the arms of a fried calamari with pasta.

    DO pick one or even two other options ahead of time, and if you haven't done this, remember your no Dry Carb rule, because there will always be another salad starter/protein or veggie entrée for you to select.

- If the restaurant lost your reservation:

    DON'T say, "Well, I tried," and pick the pizza place around the corner.

    DO try to stay calm and pick the next best option. If you steer clear of Dry Carbs and navigate the menu carefully, any restaurant will do.

- If you are tempted to make a healthy choice, overriding your true craving, and you are left unsatisfied/disappointed:

  DON'T go to the steak house, order the fish, and then eat ten ounces of your neighbor's steak. Or pick the healthy chicken at lunch and then order the BLT anyway.

  DO listen to your body. If it's a cold day and you are craving soup, don't pick the salad because you think it's healthier. Rather, choose a vegetable or chicken broth–based (not cream) soup. Or if you want the sandwich but don't want the carb (the salad just will not cut it), get the sandwich and just make dinner a clean piece of protein and a veggie. If you are at a steak house, don't order the fish (even though it will be the healthiest choice) if you really prefer the beef. Get the smallest ounce steak on the menu and order some steamed veggies and a salad to start.

- If your restaurant experience was an overall bomb:

  DON'T let it get you down.

  DO order a nice herbal or green tea or a fruit dessert. Within fifteen minutes you will be over it and you can enjoy your Fun Snack a couple of hours later.

Here are some excellent online sources for restaurant menus:

www.menupages.com Menus for many major U.S. cities.

www.menutopia.com Up-to-date restaurant menus and information for thousands of restaurants across the United States.

www.seamlessweb.com Available in many major U.S. cities as well as London. Provides menus as well as ordering services.

www.delivery.com Online food ordering from local restaurants.

ADOPT A CHEF. While sampling every great restaurant in town does have its appeal, once you've abandoned the notion of free food, your approach to business entertaining will probably change. One helpful strategy can be to pick a favorite restaurant or two to frequent when you're hosting a business meal and become a familiar face at those establishments. Many businesspeople find that there are certain restaurants that become watering holes for their industries. In New York, Michael's has long been a publishing standby and Feinstein's at the Regency Hotel is a top place for power breakfasts. Aside from the networking value, it's a diet plus to cultivate a relationship with a limited number of restaurants. You can get to know the waitstaff and the chef and indicate your dining preferences. It simplifies your dining experience when the waiter knows in advance that you prefer salads with light dressing, grilled entrées, and diet-friendly choices, and this seamless process allows you to focus entirely on business.

BEWARE THE TURKEY BURGER *Many clients tell me that they're in the habit of ordering turkey burgers. They believe they're healthier and lower in calories than a beef burger. Au contraire! A Ruby Tuesday turkey burger is roughly 812 calories with 45 grams of fat. My recommendation is to avoid turkey burgers entirely. Even when they are called "low-fat," I'm skeptical. If you enjoy turkey burgers, eat them at home where you can choose brands that you know are low in fat and calories. (See the Shopping List, page 307, for a healthy turkey burger choice.)*

OBSERVE THE ¾ RULE. The entrées in most restaurants arrive overflowing with food, and with servings that double or even triple what you should be eating. Just knowing that a portion is too large doesn't always solve the problem. Research shows that our inclination is simply to eat what's in front of us. It's important to decide in advance how to manage large portions. When your food arrives, assess the quantity on your plate and decide whether you'll eat half or three-quarters of your meal. Then stick to your decision! When you've eaten the appropriate amount, rest your knife and fork on the edge of the plate and push your plate a few inches away so that you'll be less tempted to continue nibbling and so that the waiter knows you're finished. One of my clients reported that she oversalts remaining portions when she's had enough. This keeps her from continuing to eat. There are actually two benefits to the ¾ Rule: you'll consume fewer calories and, almost as important, you'll train yourself to eat less and feel comfortable leaving food on the plate. (While you can always ask for a doggie bag of leftover food in casual dining situations, most clients tell me that they find this a bit gauche when they're entertaining. Many also avoid doggie bags because they tend to simply finish them off themselves as soon as they get home!)

CONSIDER THE APPETIZER. There is no law that says you must order a starter, an entrée, and a dessert. It's becoming quite common these days simply to order from the appetizer portion of the menu. This can guarantee smaller portions, and it can also allow you to have two courses while others are having an appetizer and an entrée. Moreover, the appetizer menu often offers an intriguing selection of choices that are as interesting as anything else on the menu. For example, in many restaurants it's not surprising to find such inviting and healthy appetizers as fresh shrimp cocktail or grilled vegetables with a light dressing. If you choose this option, you can simply tell the waiter, "I'd love to try these two appetizers and you can bring one as an appetizer and the other with the entrées." In fact, you can often divide the appetizers into very light ones that can serve as your appetizer course and more substantial appetizers that can serve as your entrée. It's best to instruct the waiter when to serve the appetizers so both of your choices won't be served at once, leaving you with nothing in front of you while the other diners are served their entrées. Here are some common appetizers divided into "starter" and "entrée" options (keep in mind that restaurant portions vary and so calorie counts here are ballpark):

Starter Options (all range from 80 to 180 calories)

- Arugula and shaved Parmesan

- Mixed greens with vinaigrette

- Beet and goat cheese salad

- Prosciutto and melon

- Asparagus vinaigrette

- Lentil soup

- 10 medium Eastern oysters

- Fresh vegetable soup

- Gazpacho

- French onion soup (no croutons, no cheese)

Entrée Options (all range from 150 to 300 calories)

- Caprese salad (buffalo mozzarella and tomato)

- Tuna tartare

- Shrimp cocktail

- Prosciutto and melon

- Steamed mussels in white wine and garlic

- Beef carpaccio

PINPOINT PRESSURE *Business is all about pressures, and one of the pressures you really don't need is the pressure to eat to excess or to eat something you'd rather skip. So let's take a clear-eyed look at the pressure points in a business meal: no one cares who eats from the bread basket, so make it a general rule to abstain. On the other hand, there can be pressure to drink alcohol and to eat dessert, so make a decision in advance how you'll handle these situations.*

MASK YOUR MOTIVES: BECOME A STEALTH DIETER. People don't like to call attention to their efforts to lose weight. Most of us have rolled our eyes when a dining companion deconstructs the menu and gives the waiter a virtual cooking course instead of an order. This is a major "diet alert" tactic and it's torture for your tablemates and your waiter to have to "hold" this and "take out" that. Just stick with a protein and the Juicy Carbs—salads and veggies. You *can* ask for double veggies; no Dry Carb. If a Dry Carb—potato, rice, etc.—lands on your plate, ignore it or oversalt it. It will soon be taken away. Of course, if you've had a chance to check the menu in advance, you'll know what to order. You'll see a list of suggestions that pertain to a variety of ethnic restaurants in the "Wall Street Cheat Sheets Restaurant Menu Survival Guide" (page 255), but my basic Wall Street generic order is a grilled protein—fish, chicken, or beef—with vegetables. That's it! Chicken is universally available, and filet mignon is a lean cut of meat and ordinarily served in reasonable portions.

Here are some more tips for Stealth Dieting:

- *Follow the One Request Rule.* Try to make only one special request of the waiter. Basically, ask to skip the Dry Carb. Life is simple!

- *Learn the language of food prep.* You know to steer away from anything fried, but there are other things that you should look out for. Grilled is good. So is steamed, baked, roasted, poached, or broiled (if no sauce is involved). Sautéed can mean extra calories from oil or butter, but it's still a good choice if you don't want any of the prior preparations. Avoid anything described as buttered, breaded, smothered, scalloped, stuffed, or creamy.

- *Don't edit sandwiches.* If the meeting buffet offers nothing but a pile of sandwiches, simply choose one, or a half of one— preferably turkey with lettuce, tomato, and mustard—and eat it! Eating only the "insides" screams Atkins and is messy. And in the end you know you'll pick at the bread anyway. If you fill up on a healthy sandwich, it's easier to skip dessert later.

- *Avoid the extras.* No one notices if you skip the bread basket, the complimentary biscotti, the chips, the passed appetizers.

- *Keep a drink in one hand* and a folded napkin or tissue or fan (if you can get away with it) in the other. You can't eat what you can't grab.

- *Skip dessert.* "I don't have a sweet tooth" is a good dodge, and the old "My doctor says I can't" will work, too. A decaf or regular skim cappuccino is a terrific sweet substitute.

- *"I already ate."* This really works. Have a healthy snack in advance: two Fiber Rich crackers and peanut butter or Babybel or Laughing Cow cheese will boost your willpower tenfold. You can then eat lightly or, if at a cocktail party, for example, not at all.

- *Wine spritzers are a diet giveaway.* And they're easy to drink quickly. Vodka with soda on the rocks is a better choice. It doesn't taste great, so you'll be happy to sip all night. And you can keep adding ice cubes and no one will realize that eventually you're drinking only water.

- *Eat slowly.* Focus on the business or friends at hand. Put your fork down at least three times in the course of the meal. There's no prize for first finisher.

- *Skip the "saint salad" entrée.* You know what this is: the "I'll just have a salad" makes you feel virtuous. But those salads are sometimes truckloads of calories. For example, a Cobb salad can cost you up to 1200 calories depending on size, dressing, and add-ons, while grilled halibut with tomatoes and asparagus is likely to be only 400 calories including the cooking oil. Moreover, a protein and vegetable are more satisfying and likely to keep late afternoon hunger pangs at bay. Research has shown that adequate protein is especially important when you're trying to lose weight. The "saint salad" may also call attention to your focus on dieting, which most of us would like to avoid in a business situation. Finally, a well-prepared grilled fish along with some interesting vegetables is a dish you may be unlikely to prepare at home, so seize the opportunity to enjoy it! After all, you can prepare a big bowl of greens for yourself anytime.

NIX NERVOUS NIBBLING *Some situations jangle our nerves. Business meetings, office parties, and other events can occasionally make us feel awkward, and it's sometimes easier to eat than to talk. Instead of munching canapés, try sipping club soda to keep your hands busy and give you a distraction while you search out someone to approach for conversation.*

GO IT ALONE. People sometimes think that sharing their weight loss goals when entertaining business associates can put valuable pressure on them to stick with their resolutions. Unfortunately, clients tell me that this approach can often backfire. The undercurrent of competitiveness that is often present in business entertaining situations can be expressed in subtle and occasionally unexpected ways. Sometimes, the confounding result is a total blowout by the end of the meal as good resolutions dissolve in a miasma of back-slapping goodwill and warm banana bread pudding with caramel sauce. While there certainly are colleagues who would be supportive while you enjoy the grilled fish and skip dessert, there are others who would be only too happy to be able to say at the end of the meal, "So much for your diet, right?" as they order an after-dinner drink for you and encourage you to enjoy every last bite of that Death-by-Chocolate. Why take the chance? Remember, not everyone you're entertaining for business is your friend. Better to go it alone and keep your weight loss goals to yourself.

"This was my third attempt at a diet. My last try was the Atkins diet where I actually gained weight. Heather's diet was simple and took into consideration my busy life. I lost nearly thirty pounds over six months and kept it off for years."
> —THOMAS LIBASSI, SENIOR MANAGING DIRECTOR, GSC GROUP

Step Two: Manage Alcohol

Alcohol can be devastating to your weight loss goals. It's the fastest way to add empty calories to your meal, and it can quickly weaken your resolve when it comes to healthy eating. The average serving of 1.5 ounces of 80-proof alcohol contains about 90 calories—before mixers are added. And some cocktails deliver a punch with the parasol: a piña colada, for example, has more calories than a Big Mac. Then there's the slow dissolve effect . . . of willpower, that is. In one study on men, researchers found that subjects who consumed alcohol had a 30 percent increase in calorie intake when they ate following drinking.* But, of course, business entertaining frequently involves alcohol. I've had clients tell me that their evening scotch is a nonnegotiable part of their daily routine. Indeed, when I began to work with Wall Street clients, I always suggested they eliminate alcohol completely to save calories. It quickly became clear to me that for many people this simply was not an option. I realized I'd have to take another approach if I wanted to help them successfully lose weight in the real world.

Whatever your personal preferences regarding alcohol, there's no doubt you need strategies to successfully manage drinking in both business and social situations while achieving your weight loss goals. So if you want to drink while entertaining for business, the strategy is to allow yourself *one* "free" drink per dinner. Remember the "one out of three" rule above? If you forgo both bread and dessert, you can indulge in two drinks. These are tips that will help you stick with these resolutions:

- Avoid mixed drinks made with high-calorie sodas, juices, and mixers. Rather, choose single-shot drinks on the rocks or wine or light beer, all of which have approximately the same number of calories. An effective strategy for some people is to simply choose a drink that is their least favorite. Many clients tell me that vodka or scotch, on the rocks or with soda, is a top choice. This is because it doesn't taste that great! You're not going to be

* Hetherington, M. M., F. Cameron, D. J. Wallis, and L. M. Pirie. "Stimulation of appetite by alcohol." *Physiol Behavior* 74(3) (October 2001):283–89.

tempted to gulp either one. Moreover, it's easy to "refresh" this drink with more ice or more soda. After a while, you're drinking only soda or water, but you always have your "camouflage" drink in hand. Here are the top Wall Street alcoholic drink picks. They all have between 80 and 100 calories. (For a complete list of alcoholic drinks, see the Cheat Sheets, pages 217–19):

- Red or white wine

- Light beer

- White wine spritzer

- Vodka or scotch and soda

■ Always order your drink *with* the meal, never before (that includes pre-dinner cocktail hours). This will keep you from moving on to a second or third glass when your food arrives. Also, alcohol that is consumed with food is metabolized more slowly and is less likely to cloud your resolve than that drink at the bar on an empty stomach. Many of my clients order a bottle of Pellegrino or other sparkling water for the table, telling the waiter that they'll put in a drink order a little later. This acknowledges that you are going to order a drink but delays it.

■ Be cautious about "diet" mixers. Many people think a rum and diet cola is a better choice than a vodka and tonic, and in terms of calories, they are right. But the fact is that the artificial sweeteners in diet mixers can usher alcohol into your bloodstream more quickly than drinks made with naturally sweetened mixers or mixers that are slightly higher in calories, like tonic. In one study, blood alcohol levels were considerably higher in subjects who had had an artifically sweetened screwdriver versus one made with natural sweeteners.*

* Wu, K. L., R. Chaikomin, S. Doran, K. L. Jones, M. Horowitz, and C. K. Rayner. "Artificially sweetened versus regular mixers increase gastric emptying and alcohol absorption." *American Journal of Medicine* 119(9) (September 2006):802–4.

- Office parties can be confusing. They might look and feel like social events, but the bottom line is that your behavior at the office holiday party can have a real effect on your career. (You do *not* want to be the topic of conversation at the water cooler the next day.) So enjoy yourself but follow the Wall Street guidelines: Snack beforehand so you don't drink on an empty stomach. If you do drink, limit yourself to two drinks, max. If food is being served, decide in advance if this will count as your dinner. If it *will* be your dinner, limit yourself to three to four napkins of food if there are circulating hors d'oeuvres, or in a buffet situation, three plates of food. And of course, if this is your dinner, no eating when you get home. If you know you'll be eating dinner later, take only one napkin (or small plate) of vegetables or lean protein. In either case, look for the low-cal choices like vegetables, shrimp, sushi, chicken skewers, etc. (See Top Hors d'Oeuvres Picks, page 226.) Take the opportunity to further your career: chat with people from other departments or people you've met only electronically. When your focus is conversation, not food, the event will be a personal success. If you're eating at home after an office party, pick a lower calorie frozen dinner (under 200 calories) and call it a night.

> Check to see if your company has an official policy on alcohol. Many people don't realize that some companies actually codify their expectations on alcohol consumption.

Sometimes you'll want to skip alcohol altogether. Here are some tips that will make this choice easier to accomplish and less obvious to your companions:

- Make it a personal policy *never* to drink at a business lunch. There's little pressure to do so these days, and you simply don't need those calories. The days of the three-martini lunch are long gone, and it's more common to skip lunchtime drinks than to indulge. Even if your companion is drinking, it's perfectly acceptable for you to skip.

- Always avoid alcohol during the day. When you have a drink in the evening, you go home and go to bed. When you drink during the day, you come down from the alcohol and feel exhausted, and this can prompt poor food choices for the rest of the day.

- Whenever possible, let others order drinks first. If iced tea seems to be the order of choice, then it's easy for you to follow suit. There's no point in ordering an alcoholic drink that you don't really want only to find that others are abstaining.

- During cocktail hours and pre-dinner drinks, sip a glass of club soda with lime (which looks enough like a mixed drink to deter questions about why you're not drinking).

- If you want to be a stealth dieter and don't want to order club soda in front of others at the bar, excuse yourself to the restroom while everyone else orders, so you can order alone later.

- Order a bottle of sparkling or mineral water at the table in a restaurant. If the waiter sees you have bottled water, you will be less pressured to order a drink.

- If possible, seek out the waiter (on the way to the restroom, for example) and ask him not to refill your wineglass or offer you additional drinks.

- Never lose track of how much you've been drinking. Sometimes a zealous waiter can rush to refill your wineglass at every opportunity. In these situations, it's easy to become fuzzy about how much you've consumed. Make it clear to the waiter that you don't want any more, or simply let your glass be filled one last time and move it out of reach so you won't be tempted to keep sipping. Alternatively, ordering something like vodka can be a good choice because the waiter will never automatically refill your drink; *you* must place the order.

> See the Wall Street Cheat Sheets (pages 217–19) for a handy list of alcoholic drinks and their calorie content.

Step Three: Take Your Time

You're accustomed to rushing. Speed is the name of your game. You want to get things done yesterday. But while you may effectively push the speed limit in your work, similar impulses at the table can turn you into a speed eater and that's the HOV lane to diet death. Many of my clients are shocked when they recognize that their habit of wolfing down deli meals at their desks has migrated to their business meals. If you're the first one to finish your meal in a restaurant, you're probably eating more than everyone else. If your plate is empty quickly, you'll be more tempted to reach for the bread basket or order dessert. It's time to put the brakes on manic munching. Here are some tips that have helped my clients reach their personal goal of being the slowest eater at the table:

- Be a talker and a listener—not an eater. The main purpose of a business meal is to build relationships and conduct business. You will eat far less, and profit more from a business standpoint, if you focus on conversation rather than on food.

- Sip water frequently between bites. This helps to fill you up, and it also creates a natural pause in the meal. Try to have the waiter refill your water glass at least three times.

- Put your utensils down at least three times in the course of a meal. Pause. Smile. Chat. Resume eating. This is the one business situation where your goal is to be last!

- Take a bathroom break at an appropriate time in the meal. Taking a break gives your brain a chance to process the fact that you may well be full. It will be easier to stop eating when you return to the table.

"I knew I was in trouble with my weight when I had to go out and buy new suits to wear to work. I literally felt uncomfortable in my own skin. I was tired all the time. I'm in my twenties and I was starting to feel old. I knew exactly what my problem was: work. Or, to be more specific, the four to five business dinners I had to attend each week. No matter how good I was all day, I'd blow it when I went out to eat. One night it would be a steak house, the next night it would be a new French restaurant. Often the dinners lasted for hours. The clients were usually in from out of town and ready for a big night. I'd arrive home totally stuffed and ready to crash from exhaustion. I think my biggest problem was wine. It's just so easy when you're entertaining to drink more than you usually would. I'm not talking about a hangover, but with cocktails, a shared bottle of wine with dinner, and a drink afterwards, the calories add up. I'd try to abstain, but then I'd find myself substituting the wine with more food.

"One of the most important things I learned from the Wall Street Diet is that one drink isn't going to do any damage. It's that second drink that starts to wear away my resistance to extra bread, rich entrées, and desserts. Just knowing I can have that one glass of wine felt so liberating, and I love Heather's strategies for sticking with my goals. By keeping my alcohol intake in check, I've been able to stick to my other dining-out resolutions, and I don't feel in the least deprived.

"I lost my extra twenty pounds in three months and ran the New York City Marathon. Three years later, I'm still running, and entertaining clients most nights of the week, but I've kept the weight off. The Wall Street Diet has become my eating lifestyle."

—NICOLE B., MERGERS AND ACQUISITIONS

Business Entertaining Off the Beaten Track

Business entertaining doesn't always mean sitting down to a five-star dinner. There are other mealtime situations that require clever strategies to help you stay on track with both your business and diet objectives.

Breakfast

Wall Street dieters love breakfast meetings. You're fresh and energetic first thing in the morning. Your resolve is strong. Healthy food choices are generally widely available. And the meeting time is usually shorter, as everyone is eager to get to the office. Many of my clients tell me they always choose a breakfast meeting when given the opportunity, for all the above reasons. Consider these breakfast meeting tips:

- Omelets—egg-white, made with Egg Beaters, or even whole eggs, with added veggies—are a good breakfast choice, but be careful to avoid regular omelets, which can be made with up to six eggs. If you'd like cheese in your omelet, ask for just one slice, otherwise they might add several pieces. Always ask for minimal butter or oil in the preparation.

- Two poached eggs with lettuce, tomato, and an order of fruit salad is a good, light breakfast choice.

- Low-fat or nonfat yogurt with berries makes a great breakfast.

- Eggs Benedict (no hollandaise sauce, English muffin = Juicy Carb) is an option.

- Eggs Florentine (no muffin, no sauce, extra spinach) is another good choice.

- Skip the granola on yogurt or as a cereal. It usually has too many calories.

- Skip fruit juice. It's generally high in calories and certainly less filling than whole fruit. Drink plain water or seltzer instead. Have a sliced orange or half a grapefruit in place of the juice.

- Canadian bacon is surprisingly low in calories and makes a good protein accompaniment.

- If you lighten your coffee or tea, always ask for skim or 2% milk. Those lovely little pitchers filled with cream add way too much fat to your morning beverage.

- Skip the pastries, croissants, pancakes, and waffles.

- Oatmeal with fruit is a good, filling morning choice. But watch the portion size: you should be having about 1 cup cooked or a fist-sized amount. Be sure it's made with water, not milk or cream.

- Cereal can be a good choice. Enjoy it with skim milk and fruit if you like. Check the Shopping List (pages 305–6) for the best brands. Of course your choices in a restaurant will be limited, but as a general rule, stick with the flakes—any type of flake cereal without added sugar or dried fruit. You can usually count on finding Special K and Cheerios, which are both good choices.

Buffets

Buffets can be a challenge, no doubt about it. There's nothing like a groaning board of endless choices to make any dieter weak in the resolve. There are three formidable factors at every buffet that research (as well as the experience of countless dieters) has shown can promote overeating: too much variety, eating with a crowd, and quickly cleared plates that remove evidence of food already consumed. It's a perfect storm for dieters. But you can conquer a buffet with these strategies:

- Don't rush to be first in the buffet line. This is one of those situations where being last can be a good thing. Walk the length of the buffet to scan what's available. It's foolish to load up on poor choices only to discover that some excellent, diet-friendly selections are available at the end of the line.

- Consider your plate. It should contain 50 percent vegetables, 25 percent carbs, and 25 percent protein. If you are having more than one drink, you should shift to 75 percent vegetables and 25 percent protein and skip the carbs entirely.

- Go for the gold. Often the less interesting and less expensive food is at the *beginning* of the buffet line. Skip the bread, the pasta salad, and any of the routine offerings. Save your appetite and calories for the better choices near the end: the lean, fresh carved meat or grilled fish. A small portion of exquisite food is a much better choice than a mountain of macaroni salad.

- Focus on greens. Choose salads and vegetables to fill your plate. Drizzle with a small amount of dressing—light dressing, if available. Select a lean protein like grilled fish, chicken, or beef.

- Consider using a small plate if there are any available. But keep in mind that sometimes a larger plate is necessary if there are good green salad choices available, as they often take up more room.

- Skip dessert. Most buffets have a separate dessert table, and sometimes it's not even set up until most people are finished with the buffet. A Wall Street dieter avoids the dessert table entirely. A dessert buffet is diet quicksand. A taste of this, a nibble of that, a few teeny tiny truffles . . . Before you know it, you're sunk up to your hips! If you know that fresh fruit is available, the best strategy is to ask someone else to grab you a plate when others are getting their own desserts. You can always substitute a cup of coffee or tea for dessert if you like.

Embrace the "Arm's Length" Rule. Wherever you are—a friend's house, an office party, a bar—always make sure you're at least an arm's length away from any food. This prevents the mindless grab and gobble and will save you many calories.

Cocktail Dinners

Cocktail dinners are cocktail parties that include dinner—or at least so much food that it counts as dinner. Sometimes it's food that's passed by strolling waiters; sometimes it's stations of various foods. You can handle a cocktail dinner occasion in two ways: You can plan to turn it into your dinner by making judicious choices. Or you can treat it as a meet-and-greet opportunity and plan to have dinner following the event. In both cases, controlling your intake of both food and alcohol when the servers seem hell-bent on filling your glass and your plate can take deft moves. Some strategies?

- Decide in advance if the gathering will serve as your dinner. If so, choose three to four napkins of food to eat.

- The One Out of Three Rule can be hard to follow at a passed dinner. In general, it's easiest to just call it a two-carb night and let it go at that. But do try to choose the healthiest passed foods, like seafood, grilled meats, and any type of vegetables.

- Keep your hands full. If you have a glass in one hand and a napkin or a handkerchief or a clutch or any decoy object in the other, it's hard to take yet another mini crab cake or baby burger from the passing tray.

- Prepare your refusals in advance: "No, thanks. I've already tried one and they're delicious." "Lovely, thanks, but I just couldn't eat one more thing."

- Focus on networking and conversation. It really isn't about the food. You'll want to look back on the event as an occasion where you met new people rather than tried new appetizers.

- Ladies should wear something fitted and men should tighten their belts a notch. It's surprising how this little trick can help keep you in check.

Some tips on tapas and Asian group dinners. In these instances you can't ordinarily make any special orders, so here are some guidelines:

- The evening counts as your carb (not counting the alcohol) because these foods tend to have sugary and starchy sauces.

- Pick only protein and vegetable choices.
- If the food comes in waves, pick only one choice on each wave. Don't be a double dipper.
- If you want to be a stealth dieter, choose something you don't like for your plate but just leave it there.
- Eat slowly and drink a lot of water, as these meals tend to be quite salty.

Restaurant Action Plan Cheat Sheet

- Plan ahead

  - Snack strategically
  - Choose two out of three: drinks, bread, dessert
  - Master the menu
  - Adopt a chef
  - Remember the ¾ Rule
  - Consider the appetizer
  - Know the Wall Street generic orders
  - Go it alone

- Manage alcohol

  - Drink alcohol only *with* the meal
  - Choose low-cal drinks
  - Avoid diet mixers
  - Manage office parties

- Take your time

  - Focus on conversation, not food
  - Drink water, at least 3 glasses
  - Rest your fork regularly
  - Take a bathroom break

The Wall Street
Travel Itinerary: Trimming
the Fat from Your
Business Trips

There's nothing like a change in the daily routine to make us feel out of sorts and inclined to overeat. And how about changing the routine and adding lots of additional stress—like increased security at airports, delayed flights, pressure to perform in a new setting, unfamiliar cities, poor food choices, and a TV remote with buttons in the wrong places? From those first moments running through the airport at a hideously early hour, searching for something, anything, to call breakfast, to that last frustrating and seemingly endless pause waiting for an open gate for the plane, travel can be a binge-inducing glitch waiting to happen. It's enough to drive many of us to despair and to the minibar. Because what is there, after all, to comfort us when we're away from friends and family and our own familiar world? Well, how about a Cinnabon and a mocha frappacino? Yes, for many of us, food is a great comforter. If, in the past, you've allowed the common business travel side effects of boredom, fatigue, frustration, and general stress to translate into hunger and overindulgence, I'll show you how to manage them and come home lean and light.

The physical stresses of travel can certainly drive you to eat. But sometimes there's an additional, more subtle issue to cope with: an undercurrent of resentment that business travelers pack along with their laptops. After all, when you travel for work, you're working twenty-four hours a day. You're away from the things you love, and you're enduring hardships. Yes, a first class seat, luxury hotel, free stationery, and a breakfast buffet can be nice, but, as Dorothy told Auntie Em, "There's no place like home." So what do you do with this barely buried resentment? You feed it. After all, you deserve a reward. You're a road warrior. A hungry, lonely, bored, tired road warrior.

But you know the sad truth about business travel: what happens in the hotel *doesn't* stay in the hotel. It follows you home and shows up on your scale. If regular or even occasional business travel is part of your lifestyle, you need a plan—a set of strategies that will ensure you eat as healthfully on the road as you do at home. You need to consider both the physical stresses and the psychological stresses that trigger overeating. The bottom line of business travel is performance, and here's where you'll learn how to manage your diet so that your energy levels and your overall performance will be top-notch—whether you're flying first class or hopping in and out of your minivan.

"It wasn't until I started to travel for business that I began to gain weight. I'd sleep restlessly the night before I had to go somewhere. Then I'd feel tired and wound up as I headed—usually at the crack of dawn—to the airport. I'd grab a giant coffee and maybe a Danish or bagel with cream cheese before the flight. Then I'd eat absolutely everything they served on the flight, even if I didn't like it. I felt like I 'needed' it and 'deserved' it. From that point on, I'd eat poorly until I got home. When I traveled, my schedule always felt out of whack. I was tired all the time. I wasn't getting any exercise, and for some reason I always felt like food was going to make me feel better. Of course it never did, and I invariably got home exhausted, frazzled, and with a food hangover as well as a few extra pounds. But the Wall Street Diet has completely transformed my business trips. It's hard for me to believe that just thinking differently about the trip and using certain tips on what to eat and how to snack can make such a difference. It's not just that I eat better and that I've lost weight. The bottom line is that I feel like a totally different person. No matter

where I am in the world, my energy level is high and I feel in control. To be honest, that means as much to me as the weight loss. My family has noticed the difference, too. It used to take me a day or two to recover from a business trip. Now I find, even if I'm a little tired, that I can hit the ground running the minute I get back from a trip. Sometimes I do a Protein Day; other times I just go right back to my daily routine. Either way, I've lost the weight I needed to lose, and in three years I haven't gained any back."

—DAN S., PARTNER, MAJOR MANHATTAN LAW FIRM

The overriding theme of successful Wall Street business trips is control—of your choices, your healthy routine, and most important, your food intake. Too many people find themselves thinking of everything but food when they prepare for a trip, and this can leave them vulnerable to energy lows and poor choices as they make their way through the maze of airports and taxis and hotels.

The trick is to *know yourself* and eat the least amount of food you need to feel satisfied and energetic.

Set up your trip to meet your health goals. I'll explain how to achieve this by turning your business trip into a spa trip. I'll show you how to choose your hotel, your airport foods, and your meals on the road as a seamless part of your diet, not an interruption to your healthy lifestyle. For you, this could mean a breakfast that consists of a simple skim venti latte in the airport followed by a healthy lunch three or four hours later. For others, it could be a coffee plus fruit and low-fat yogurt with half a granola bar (which crumbles well) mixed into it. Perhaps a hotel with a jogging trail will make all the difference to you. Maybe a hotel pool will allow you to recharge, de-stress, and burn calories. When you know what your body needs, and you plan in advance, you'll travel well and successfully and your trip will enhance, not ruin, your diet.

Let's take a look at some of the pitfalls of business travel and the foolproof strategies that will put them in your rearview mirror.

Wall Street Flight Plan

Before you even leave home on a business trip, it's a good idea to run through your travel plans and assess how they'll affect your meals and snacks. Consider the following issues:

WHAT WILL YOU EAT EN ROUTE? If you're flying, what food will be served on your flight and do you plan to eat it? This will determine whether or not you need to provide your own travel meal and snacks. Most people can quickly check online before they leave home—usually when they print their boarding pass—about the meal situation. If you're flying first class, you will probably be served food. Some people will not eat airline food and they have to be prepared with their own snacks and meals. Others—usually Clean Plate Clubbers—will eat whatever is put in front of them, and they need strategies to limit their intake.

> *I have a client who uses her flights as a "cleanse." She tells the attendants that she wants only hot water and lemon during the flight; no food. She reports that she feels light and fantastic when she disembarks.*

If you're traveling by car or train, it's easier to manage your meals and snacks. You can pack meals and snacks in a cooler in the car, or if you're going by train, you can take along almost any foods you can carry. Road trips usually mean food stops, and these can be surprisingly healthy interludes. My best advice here is to avoid highway rest stops, which can often be time-consuming and which offer limited choices. Look for the fork in the road (those signs that indicate that food is available off the next exit). Exit and look for a Subway. Subways are easy to find and now offer a line of healthy meals called Subway Fresh Fit Meals, which include a sandwich, a fruit, and a bottle of water. You can get a veggie or turkey sandwich on this meal for between 200 and 300 calories. If you do find yourself at a highway rest stop, don't despair. You can get a healthy meal at countless fast-food places these days. For a complete list, see "High-dividend Chain Choices," page 237; but just for example, at McDonald's you can choose an Asian Salad with Grilled Chicken with Low-Fat Balsamic Vinaigrette for 340 calories, or at Taco Bell, a Ranchero Chicken Soft Taco ("Fresco Style") for 170 calories.

HOW LONG WILL YOU BE AWAY FROM HOME? If it's a day trip, you may need to plan only for an airport breakfast and/or snack. If, on the other hand, it's an overnight or multi-night trip, you'll do better if you're fully prepared. When considering air travel, keep in mind that flight time is not the same as travel time: sometimes a two-hour flight can actually mean five hours of travel when you figure in airport transport, waiting for baggage, etc. I always advise clients that a longer trip requires a travel food pack. This should include the appropriate number of energy bars as well as other snacks of your choice.

WHAT'S YOUR DAILY SCHEDULE WHILE AWAY? Do you have just one or two meetings a day? Or is virtually every minute of your time away accounted for with meetings and business entertaining? This will determine how many snacks you'll want to pack and also how much advance research you might want to do on local restaurants as well as potential exercise options.

Once you've assessed what's ahead of you on any particular trip, you've won half the battle. But it's also helpful to consider some of the challenges you'll face in choosing meals and snacks on the road. And I have some extremely useful suggestions for booking hotels, working out on the road, and conquering that shaky reentry period when you're just back from a trip.

Terminal Breakfast

It does feel terminal, doesn't it? You're so hungry that you've already forgotten your gate number three times. You left home in a frantic rush, with nothing but the taste of toothpaste in your mouth. And now, nearly two hours later, you realize that they're not serving a meal on your flight and it could be late afternoon before you actually have access to a meal. What to do? At first glance, airport breakfast offerings seem totally discouraging. There are the giant wheels of frosted or unfrosted carbs or . . . well, that seems to be about it. Don't despair. There are terrific breakfast options available at every airport—really quick, healthy grab-and-go early-morning meals—and they'll emerge like Waldo from the kiosks and airport storefronts when you know where to look.

Instant Airport Breakfasts

You have ten minutes before your flight boards and before you become a victim of the rubber-egg-and-sausage assault. But all you see around you are big fat bagels larded with cream cheese and tire-sized Cinnabons. Confusion is the enemy of control, so here's how to keep it simple and choose a healthy, light, satisfying breakfast that won't take more than ten minutes to gather. Countless clients have told me that this one-stop breakfast has saved their diet lives. There's also a two-stop breakfast for those who have a bit more time and/or want a bit more food.

ONE-STOP BREAKFAST. Dash into Starbucks or any coffee shop for a venti skim latte. Yes, it really is half of a healthy breakfast. It's a shot of espresso along with roughly 9 ounces of milk that will cost you about 200 calories. You can get it with skim or soy milk. The soy milk has a bit more sugar in it, but it's still a good choice. The second half of the one-stop breakfast is a piece of fruit. They'll have a banana or some other fruit available at almost any Starbucks or coffee shop. Some people rely on this as their standard airport breakfast even if they have a bit of extra time, particularly if they've packed a healthy snack for the plane ride. I never used to recommend a venti breakfast to others, even though I relied on it myself, because it didn't seem healthy enough. After all, coffee for breakfast is not a nutritionist's dream. But if you're trying to lose weight, and you're in a mad rush, a nice drink of milk and a piece of fruit, which will fill you up and sustain you for a few hours, is a perfectly fine way to start your day. Another plus to a venti skim latte if you're a woman is that it provides roughly 60 percent of your RDA for calcium.

THE TWO-STOP BREAKFAST. Have a few more minutes? Looking for a more substantial breakfast? Do your Starbucks run for tea or coffee. While you're there, pick up a non- or low-fat yogurt (e.g., Dannon Light & Fit, Stonyfield Farm) and/or a piece of fruit, depending on whether you're a man or a woman. (See Menu guidelines below.) Your second stop is at Hudson News. Hudson News, that familiar newsstand-plus-sundries shop that you'll find in almost every airport in the country, is open at the crack of dawn and sometimes even before. There you will find a choice of energy bars that, added to your venti or tea, yogurt, and fruit, will provide protein and fiber and will fill you up.

TWO-STOP BREAKFAST MENU. Women should choose one or two of the following; men, two or three:

- Non- or low-fat yogurt (e.g., Dannon Light & Fit, Stonyfield Farm)

- Fruit like a banana or an orange*

- Energy bar

By the way, if you're choosing an energy bar in the morning, I suggest you avoid any with chocolate as it sends the wrong food message to your brain; stick with the plainer bars for breakfast. My top energy bar breakfast picks (available at Hudson News) are:

- Nature Valley granola bar

- Balance bar

- South Beach bar

- Soy Joy bar

- PowerBar Harvest (a bit high in calories at 250 but acceptable)

*"Covered" fruit that you don't have to wash is best.

Most travelers are aware that the Transportation Security Administration (TSA) has instituted strict regulations about the amount of toothpaste, bottled water, and other liquid and gel items permitted in carry-on luggage. Most recent regulations prohibit liquids and gels in excess of three ounces through airport security, but snacks like bananas, apples, fresh-cut veggies, energy bars, etc., are currently acceptable. When you've passed through security, you can buy bottled water for the flight. Check with your carrier online before your flight to be sure you're up-to-date on the most recent regulations. In general, it's safest to buy carry-on foods like salads and sandwiches after you've cleared security.

This Two-stop Breakfast is a healthy, light meal that provides some protein and fiber while it fills you up. Of course you'll have to use your common sense. If you know you're going to be fed on the flight and you know you're going to eat the breakfast that's served and you know you'll have that meal within an hour or so, you would do better to simply have tea or coffee in the airport.

If, however, you are looking for something more to eat than a One- or Two-stop Breakfast, there are options. I've provided some good choices in the Airport Cheat Sheets (page 262), but a few quick ideas include a McDonald's Egg McMuffin with the bread removed, the Burger King Egg, Ham & Cheese Sandwich without the bread, or the Au Bon Pain arugula and tomato or ham and cheddar frittata.

> *"Here's what I like about the Wall Street airport food suggestions: I don't have to think about food anymore when I travel. I do the Two-stop Breakfast when I travel early. I always have my food carry-ons. I can purchase either of my two favorite healthy fast foods anywhere when I need to. Everything is automatic. It's relaxing and efficient and I've kept the weight off even when I'm traveling constantly."*
>
> —THOMAS K., GALLERY OWNER

Flying Snacks

So you're cruising along at thirty thousand feet. You had your skim latte two hours ago in the airport, but then the flight sat at the gate forever, and you're not going to get a real meal for hours. And you're hungry! But wait . . . here comes an airline snack pack. And it would be oh so welcome if it were anything but a salty, calorie-laden fat bomb. Why does an airline think a nine-hundred-calorie carb festival that includes a bag of pretzels, a mini box of cheese with crackers, and a brownie is a snack? The worst of this situation is that your resistance is extremely low: you're hungry, you're probably tired, and you've been reduced to that infantile feed-me mentality that most of us adopt the minute we fasten our seat belts.

The solution to this is to never, ever board a flight without one or two healthy snacks. (Passport? Check. Laptop? Check. Healthy snack? Check.) Many of my clients like to grab a skim latte before they board the flight, but they also want to have something to eat later. In some cases, they don't eat airline food at all and so will decline any breakfast that's served. In other cases, they're on a flight that doesn't serve any food. Some people like to take along carry-on food as insurance against flight delays, missed connections, or even just to stash in their hotel room fridge on arrival and have on hand for the return flight, just in case. I've found that some men, in particular, like to have a meal-shake option to keep in their briefcases.

> Fiber Rich crackers fit perfectly into plastic travel soap containers, and many of my clients keep one always stocked in their briefcase.

Before you toss a batch of snacks into your briefcase, you have to recognize what you can handle having aboard. My clients always can answer this question: they know that either they can have extra snacks on board or, particularly if they're CPCers, they can't because they'll simply eat whatever they carry. The best Clean Plate Club snacks are Babybel Light cheeses (one of my clients calls them "the indestructible cheese") and Fiber Rich crackers. If you're a CPC person on a longer trip, it's safer to pack any extra snacks in your checked or stowed luggage; you should keep just enough food for the actual flight within handy access. If you're a Controlled Eater, you can pack whatever snacks you like from the suggested list below. The bars and cheese/cracker snacks will come in handy in hotel rooms, extended meetings, before business dinners and cocktail parties, and in delayed-flight situations. Consider taking along some peanut butter tubes to have with your crackers. In addition, you might want to take along tea bags, as most hotel rooms have the facilities to heat water. A cup of tea in the evening can subvert cravings and relax you at the same time. If you're totally on the run on the way to your flight, you can at least pick up an energy bar at Hudson News or any other airport shop. (See the Wall Street bar picks, page 150.) Remember that sometimes on a flight you're really not hungry; you're thirsty. So drink water or club soda or tea at every opportunity.

THE WALL STREET EMERGENCY SNACK PACK *I suggest that clients who travel for work always take along an Emergency Snack Pack. Your Emergency Pack should include: 1 bar or shake, 2–4 Fiber Rich crackers, and either 1 tube of peanut butter or 2 Babybel Light cheeses. (The advantage of peanut butter is that it doesn't require refrigeration and can stay in the bag indefinitely; the cheese should be fresh for each trip.)*

Here are the recommended Wall Street Flying Snacks that will tide you over no matter what the airline or the weather dishes out:

- **WATER.** Always pick up a liter bottle before boarding your flight.

- **FRUIT/VEGGIES.** Either cut-up veggies, a piece of fruit, Crispy Delite fruit or veggie chips, Nature Valley Fruit Crisps.

- **SWEETS.** Any energy bar (without chocolate coating so it doesn't melt) such as Luna toasted nuts and cranberry, Balance honey yogurt, Kashi TLC granola bar, Lärabar, Gnu Foods bar.

- **CRUNCHY/SALTY.** Glenny's Soy Crisps, Boston's Lite all-natural popcorn (60-calorie bag), Glenny's Zen tortilla chips.

- **PROTEIN-PACKED.** Justin's nut butter and 2 Fiber Rich Crackers; 2 mini Babybel Light or Laughing Cow Light and 2 Fiber Rich; Shelton's free-range turkey jerky (50-calorie bag) and 2 Fiber Rich; Laughing Cow Cheese & Baguettes (60 calories).

- **QUICK FIX.** Ready-to-drink nonrefrigerated shakes (ask for a cup with ice once you're on the plane), Myoplex Lite shake (190 calories), Myoplex Carb Sense shake (150 calories).

See the Shopping List, pages 304–315, for some details about the above products.

FLYING TRAVEL TIP *Always save any food you've taken on board a flight until the airline meal or snack is served. Serve yourself when the flight attendants serve others. Otherwise it's too easy to eat your own meal or snack and also eat what the airline provides.*

ACTUAL AIRLINE MEALS. In-flight meals are the Rodney Dangerfields of food: they don't get no respect. Back in the day, they were a joke because of the overall poor quality of what was offered. Today they're a joke because, on many flights, they've disappeared. In fact, the story of airline food is summarized in the old joke: "The food was terrible. And the portions were way too small." What's a traveler to do? There are steps you can take to improve your lot when it comes to eating aloft. First, you should always check with the airlines to see what food, if any, will be served on your flight. If a meal is served aboard and you are going to eat it, here's how to turn it into a Wall Street Meal: eat the vegetables, protein, salad, and fruit, and skip the Dry Carbs, including the bread, potato, rice, pasta, and dessert. Because airline portions are so small, if you follow this advice, you'll be eating a relatively low-calorie, healthy meal. If nothing will be served, see pages 153–54 for carry-on food suggestions. And by the way, if you want to skip the meal entirely, let the flight attendant know in advance that you don't want to be disturbed on the flight. I have clients who do this regularly and thus are never tempted by anything the airline dishes out.

HYDRATE! *You certainly aren't going to carry a case of water bottles on a flight, but be sure you have at least one small water bottle on your person at all times. Travel, particularly plane travel, is dehydrating, and your access to fresh water may be limited. The Wall Street goal is to consume 32 ounces of water on a flight (unless it's a brief shuttle flight!).*

FLYING FLUIDS. You know you need to hydrate while flying. The dry cabin air and the distraction of travel can leave you parched. And dehydration can make you feel foggy and less able to make smart food choices. It's also healthy to drink sufficient fluids, as a good fluid intake insures frequent strolls to the bathroom to stretch your legs. The best basic fluid choice is, of course, water. Pick up a bottle in the terminal (after clearing security) if you can so you can sip from the moment you're in your seat. Sometimes it takes a while before you're offered a drink, if you're offered anything at all, on the flight. If you like, take along some Crystal Light packets (many newsstands sell them right next to the water) to add flavor to your bottled water. If you have a choice of beverages on your flight, choose water, tea, seltzer, or a juice spritzer (seltzer with a splash of fruit juice). Avoid alcohol entirely while flying. It can promote dehydration and can also be the first step in undoing all your good intentions. Also avoid a Virgin Mary. Many clients told me that they thought this was a good beverage choice, but it's far too high in sodium (a 12-ounce Mr. & Mrs. T Bloody Mary Mix has 2100 mg of sodium!) and can promote dehydration and also make those high-cal, salty, airline snacks even more appealing.

> If you tend to get stomach upset while flying, avoid beverages like coffee, alcohol, and orange juice, which are known to irritate the stomach. Instead, ask for drinks like club soda or herb tea, which seem to soothe the gastrointestinal tract. Remember that alcohol can hit you much harder at three thousand feet than in your local watering hole. It's best to avoid alcohol entirely when traveling.

Traveling Lunches and Dinners

What's your lunch plan? Will you be traveling during lunchtime? Will you be served a healthy lunch on the flight? Are you on a road trip that will involve a pit-stop lunch? Or are you traveling later in the day, when you may need to be eating dinner on the road or in the airport?

Here are some lunch and dinner solutions:

PACK YOUR OWN. If you have the time and supplies, this is a great solution. You'll know what you're getting and you can suit yourself in terms of choices and calories. Although this approach can often be an excellent nutritional strategy, the truth is my clients rarely take the time to do this. But if you do have the time, particularly if you're on a road trip and can make use of a cooler, pack up a turkey sandwich on a La Tortilla wrap or light whole wheat bread, with mustard and lots of chopped lettuce. This is a terrific, tasty, diet-friendly sandwich. Toss some baby carrots in a Ziploc bag and grab some Babybel or Laughing Cow Light cheeses and Fiber Rich crackers and you're good to go. This selection of food will definitely get you through until dinnertime.

AIRPORT LUNCH AND DINNER CHOICES. You really can get a decent meal in an airport. You just have to choose wisely. Your best general choice if searching for a meal is a salad. You can find a grilled chicken Caesar salad almost anywhere. Most times they'll be served without dressing, but if not, you can always request dressing on the side. Choose one with a light Italian or vinaigrette or a fat-free dressing, or if none of these are available, dress it yourself with a little drizzle of oil and vinegar from the salad bar. Request no croutons on the salad if possible; if that's not possible, pick them off. Sandwiches can also be great lunch choices. Many people, especially Veteran Dieters, are wary of the carbs in a sandwich, but in fact, other choices, like fruit and nut mixes, that people try to make a meal of are actually poor choices compared to a sandwich, because they are not as satisfying and they can contribute to spikes and dips in blood sugar and thus promote fatigue. Starbucks offers premade sandwiches that have the calorie count listed on the package. Look for their choices under 350 calories, such as their turkey and Swiss sandwich at 280 calories with no condiments or their Very Veggie Crunch Wrap for 310 calories. The ideal Wall Street sandwich is turkey, lettuce, and tomato on whole wheat bread with mustard. It's delicious, filling, and available almost anywhere. Don't hesitate to ask any airport restaurant, even a chain restaurant, to make it to your order. Alternatively, you can always ask for steamed vegetables and some kind of grilled protein and request that they hold the Dry Carbs (French fries, pasta, rice, baked potato).

> FLIGHT DELAYED? CANCELED? *If you learn that you have hours to kill before you can get on a flight, consider checking out* airportgyms.com *to see what gym facilities are in or nearby the terminal. This handy site lists gyms and their amenities in most major U.S. and Canadian airports as well as nearby facilities, their amenities, fees if any, and the cost of transport to them (which sometimes is a free shuttle). A five-hour delay could mean a great workout, a steam, and a shower rather than a frustrating time-killer.*

For many of my clients, it's been a major breakthrough to learn that fast-food restaurants as well as chain restaurants offer some excellent meal choices these days. Many people have told me that they've wandered airport terminals, starving, searching for healthy meals, and given up because all they could find was a McDonald's and a Chili's, which they believed were diet death traps. While it's true that many chain and fast-food restaurants are diet minefields, it's also true that, when you know where to look, you can get a healthy, satisfying meal on a tray at almost any airport in the country.

Here are some top Wall Street terminal chain lunch or dinner picks (check the Cheat Sheets, page 262, for a complete list of airport terminal choices):

Au Bon Pain Picks and Skips

PICK	CALORIES
Southwest vegetable soup (medium)	100
Thai chicken salad	190
With fat-free raspberry vinaigrette (80)	270
Caesar salad	210
With fat-free raspberry vinaigrette (80)	290

SKIP	CALORIES
Shanghai Salad (with Asian sesame dressing)	980
Turkey melt	1030

Burger King Picks and Skips

PICK	CALORIES
Side garden salad	15
With Ken's fat-free ranch dressing (60)	75
Hamburger (without the bun)	160
Hamburger	290
TenderGrill chicken garden salad (without dressing)	240
With Ken's fat-free ranch dressing (60)	300

SKIP	CALORIES
Triple Whopper sandwich	1130
BK Quad Stacker	1000

McDonald's Picks and Skips

PICK	CALORIES
Side garden salad	20
With low-fat balsamic vinaigrette (40)	60
Hamburger (without the bun)	90
Fruit and walnut salad (snack-sized)	210
Hamburger	250
Caesar salad with grilled chicken	220
With low-fat balsamic vinaigrette (40)	260
Honey Mustard Snack Wrap	
(grilled chicken)	260
Asian salad with grilled chicken	300
With low-fat balsamic vinaigrette (40)	340

SKIP	CALORIES
Double Quarter Pounder with Cheese	740
With medium French fries (380)	1120
Premium Crispy Chicken Club Sandwich	660

There's one last iron-clad Wall Street rule when it comes to in-flight eating: never eat alone! That is, never eat unless the cart has reached you and is serving other passengers. Begin your meal or snack when the cart is in your aisle; never before. Too many people find that they eat their snack or meal on takeoff, thinking that they'll work or nap or read afterward, only to find that once that cart reaches them, they are eating a second meal or snack. So make it easy on yourself; the serving cart is your signal to begin your own healthy meal.

Spa Trip: A Whole New Way to Travel

Life on the road can be challenging. There are the odd hours, the
strange bed, the disrupted mealtimes. And of course there's the whole
point of business travel: doing business! You must be focused and you
must perform at appropriate times. So yes, it's demanding and often tir-
ing and stressful. But let's take a look at the *opportunities* of business
travel. You are free of household responsibilities. You can jump out of
bed, brush your teeth, and go: no bed to make, no dog to walk, no cat to
feed. No shopping, cooking, or bills to pay. No partner or family to
please.

The Wall Street philosophy is that you have two lives—your personal life and your business life—and all reasonable indulgences should
be reserved for your personal life. That means no chocolate bar because
you're bored in the hotel room, no big dessert after a business dinner, no
logging in another half hour of sleep when you could be in the hotel gym
getting a head start on your day. Enjoy a hot dog at the ball game with
your child, a fancy drink with your friends at a celebratory dinner, and
an extra morning snooze on your personal time. Keep work time lean
and clean. Use this mentality to turn every business trip into a spa inter-
lude. Get your work done, exercise, eat light, and come home refreshed.
Once you change your mind-set about business travel, you'll find that
you can look forward to a business trip as a healthy respite from your
daily routine.

Here are some Wall Street Spa Trip tips:

CHOOSE YOUR HOTEL CAREFULLY. Business customers are important
to hotels, and they want you to be happy. These days, many hotels cater-

ing to business travelers offer amenities that will make your stay both more pleasant and healthier. Always try to choose a hotel that has a fitness center and, if you swim, a pool. Some Internet booking sites, including Travelocity and Orbitz, allow you to customize your hotel search to select hotels that offer these facilities. Some hotels also offer "light and fit" options on their room service menus, and while this option might not be sufficient reason to choose a certain hotel, it's certainly something to look for once you've checked in. If you travel regularly to the same cities, find a hotel that meets your needs and stick with it. Repeat customers often enjoy extra benefits, and it makes the whole travel process smoother and easier.

CUSTOMIZE YOUR ROOM. It's midnight and you just got back to your hotel room following an endless business dinner that capped an endless strategy meeting. You've never been more exhausted. You flip on the news, peel off your shoes, and then . . . what's that sound? It's the sweet, siren call of a tiny fridge filled with Toblerone chocolates, giant Twix bars, and "gourmet" nut mixes. The midnight song of the minibar has led too many travelers astray. For any Wall Street Dieter, but particularly for Clean Plate Club Eaters, one of the most important calls you can make before you leave home is the one asking the hotel to clear the minibar in your room. Hotels are happy to do this with advance warning. Sometimes there's a nominal fee, but in any event, the small fee is no doubt less than what you might spend on the Cadbury bars. You can use the extra space in the little fridge for water, fruit, or other healthy snacks.

FASTEN YOUR SEAT BELTS . . . *Fatigue often masquerades as hunger. You think you're hungry, but you're actually tired. This is a major travel consideration because your normal sleeping and eating routines are interrupted. It helps to remind yourself that you may well be tired, not hungry. Don't compound the negative effects of fatigue by mindless eating.*

PACK YOUR GYM. While I doubt you're going to want to haul along hand weights in your luggage, I suggest you *always* pack your sneakers and workout clothes. Some clients like to take a resistance band with them or a jump rope. Both of these make exercising in your room at your convenience a snap. Another handy option is downloading an exercise program onto your MP3 player. iTRAIN offers downloadable exercise programs for your MP3 or iPod, with choices that range from beginners' workouts to total-body boot-camp selections. You can also use the DVD on your laptop for Pilates, yoga, or other fitness CDs. If you're a walker or runner be sure to check the weather at your destination before you leave (*weather.com* provides forecasts) so you can pack the appropriate outdoor workout wear.

> *Salads are always a prime Wall Street meal option because they're low-cal and packed with nutrition. But if you're traveling in a developing country where you can risk food- or water-borne illness, skip the raw vegetable salads and stick with cooked vegetables served piping hot. Choose your drinking water carefully and ask at your hotel about water safety.*

RESET YOUR HEALTH CLOCK. You get off a plane, find your luggage, wedge it into a cab, and before you know it you're standing bleary-eyed in the center of a strange hotel room. Many clients have told me that this is a "diet pressure point" for them. The impulse is to eat. The tempting fantasy begins with a zip into the hotel convenience store for a few candy bars or a bag of chips, followed by a relaxing channel surf and then perhaps a nap in your room. This is not the best way to begin your trip, as the sugar and carbs will give you rebound fatigue and you'll have trouble with your energy levels going forward.

> *Jet lag can be a serious diet challenge. It can cause fatigue, headache, disorientation, and insomnia, and can prompt you to overindulge. Some strategies to reduce the effects of jet lag include: staying hydrated at all times while traveling, adjusting your bedtime to the local time as quickly as possible, spending some time each day out of doors (the sun will help reset your body clock), and timing your meals to the timing of local meals.*

When you're tired and foggy and you've just gotten off a flight, you often crave carbs and sugar. This is a particular issue for people who travel abroad and may also be grappling with jet lag. The deadly combination of fatigue and disorientation can result in a major, if nearly unconscious, calorie upload. In fact, research shows that sleep deprivation can promote hunger. So save yourself with a health clock reset. The simple reset formula? Sweat followed by a shower. This will dispel the fog of travel, reenergize you, and banish thoughts of snacking. You may still have to cope with jet lag, but you will feel so much better than if you'd had a snack, or a few snacks, and a nap.

Sometimes time is short after arrival at your destination. Maybe you have only an hour between hotel check-in and a meeting. If this is the case, simply stretch (or jump rope or do some sit-ups or jumping jacks) to get warmed up, and then take a long, relaxing shower. Drink plenty of water and be on your way. If you have more time, do twenty to thirty minutes of cardio at the hotel gym (even if it's on an ancient exercise bicycle) or in your room. Again, follow this with a shower and you'll be ready to face the world, and carbs and sugar cravings will be banished.

> *Looking for a healthy meal in a new city? Check out this website:* http://www.healthydiningfinder.com/site/. *Right now it seems to be heavily weighted toward chain restaurants, but sometimes even that's a help. It does have more complete listings for cities.*

EATING AT YOUR "SPA" HOTEL. You can turn almost any hotel dining room into your own personal spa. Many hotels are making a concerted effort to offer healthier choices on their menus. Even if the hotel doesn't have a healthy choice, you can create one by ordering judiciously. Use the room service menu as a basic blueprint to healthy meals. If you know there will be a breakfast buffet with poor choices, order an egg-white omelet with veggies, or oatmeal (or yogurt) with fruit, to be sent to your room. If you're expected to show up at the breakfast buffet later, you can simply enjoy some coffee or tea or perhaps some more fruit. Most hotels these days have a good selection of healthy dinners on their room service menu. You can almost always find a salad with grilled chicken or fish. Order one with dressing on the side and some fruit, and you have an excellent, healthy meal. A tip: When room service delivers the meal, the dressing usually comes in a boat. And there's normally a mound of bread. Ask the waiter to wait for a minute and take only the dressing you need and send the rest, along with the bread, back. It's just too tempting to dip that bread in the dressing once you're in your PJs and working the remote. For more suggestions on top pick Wall Street menu selections, see the Wall Street Restaurant Menu Survival Guide (page 255).

GYMS ON THE GO. *If you belong to a gym, check to see if it has affiliations with any gyms at your destination. Many gym chains participate in what's called a passport program that gives you the option of visiting gyms in other cities for free or for a nominal cost. You can check this out at passport.com. You can also check with your at-home gym to see if they have sister facilities in other cities.*

WORK IN YOUR WORKOUTS. You've already made a point to choose a hotel with exercise facilities. Now make sure you use them! Try to set up your workout schedule in your mind before you leave home, and stick with it. Your first priority is to work out first thing in the morning. It's just too hard to leave it until later in the day. Early-morning exercise will rev up your day and give you a sense of control that lasts until evening. Don't think you can catch some extra winks; that's a personal indulgence and you're in spa mode! If you wake up, exercise, shower, and grab a healthy breakfast, you'll feel ten times ahead of everyone else. As soon as you arrive at the hotel, check out the gym hours and ask the concierge or front desk about any local running or walking trails. Many hotels provide upon request custom maps that indicate safe, distance-marked routes close to the hotel. If you prefer the hotel gym, try to get there early. Take advantage of a wake-up call to prod you out of bed.

PREPARE FOR DEPARTURE. You will face the same airport issues the day of your departure, but you won't have home-court advantage: you won't be able to toss some snacks from your fridge into your briefcase. Many of my clients think ahead and bring along sufficient snacks—particularly Fiber Rich crackers and little cheeses—to get them through their trip home. But if you haven't been able to do that or if you've run out of snacks, ask the concierge for the location of the nearest local upscale grocery store and stock up on snacks to enjoy during your stay and on your trip home. Keep them in your hotel room fridge as necessary. You might also try a tactic that some of my clients have used with great success: if you have an early flight, order a breakfast to be served in your room and request that, along with the breakfast, the hotel also deliver a healthy lunch that you can take to the airport. So the night before, you might put in an order for an egg-white veggie omelet or oatmeal with fruit and also a turkey sandwich on whole wheat with mustard, lettuce, and tomato and a piece of fruit. Ask if they will package the lunch appropriately for you to take along on your trip. This tactic can save you time and frustration in the airport and can guarantee that you have at least one healthy meal for your journey home.

Reentry

Those first moments home following a business trip are often bittersweet. You're usually tired and a bit disoriented. It's wonderful to be home, but the honest truth is that your head may still be in seat 4B of flight 112. Those at home are eager to reconnect with you, but you may be tired and not quite yourself. Indeed, fatigue can make you feel like you've just had three martinis: your resistance is down and it's very hard to avoid poor food choices and mindless eating, particularly carb loading. It's important to remember: you're not hungry, you're tired. It's time to coddle yourself a bit, but not with food. Here's how:

- Take a shower or a relaxing bath.

- Get back to your at-home meal schedule. If you've missed a meal—say, dinner—in the course of your travels, have a simple dinner after your shower or bath. A frozen dinner is a good choice (see Wall Street Shopping List Frozen Meals, pages 313–14, for the top frozen dinner picks) because it's fast and portion-controlled and takes no prep. If you don't want to do a frozen dinner, figure out which restaurant will give you a nice take-out meal of a grilled protein and steamed vegetables; or if someone is at home, see if they can leave a plate of same in the fridge for you. If you have eaten on your trip, don't snack once you're home.

- Go to bed on time.

- Follow up the trip with a Protein Day. A Protein Day can save you from any inclination to binge on carbs in an unconscious effort to remedy lingering tiredness.

Wall Street Food Flight Cheat Sheet

Remember, eat only when food is served to others by flight attendants.

For flights between 1 and 3 hours, choose one of the following:

- Crunchy choices:
  - 1.3-oz bag of Glenny's Soy Crisps
  - Nature Valley Apple Fruit Crisps
  - Glenny's Zen Tortilla Chips
  - Nabisco 100-calorie snack option
  - Crispy Delite Veggie Chips

- Sweet choice:
  - Any Wall Street recommended bar (pages 311–12)

- Fruit choice:

  - Apple, orange, or small banana

- Cheese choice:

  - 2 Fiber Rich crackers plus 2 Babybel cheeses (or Laughing Cow Light)

For flights over 4 hours, choose one meal and one snack (snacks listed above):

- Wall Street breakfast:

  - Terminal Two-stop Breakfast: skim latte plus energy bar, yogurt, fruit (two for women; three for men)
  - Carry-on Breakfast: 1 packet of peanut butter squeeze with 2 Fiber Rich crackers or 1 cup dry cereal in Baggie (add skim milk from flight attendant) plus one fruit

- Carry-on Lunch or Dinner:

  - Turkey sandwich on wheat or rye with lettuce, tomato, and mustard or prepackaged salad with protein (chicken, plain tuna) and fruit (when meal cart comes around)

For long haul flights, generally over 6 hours, same as above but come prepared with breakfast, lunch, and a snack.

> *"The Wall Street Diet offers sound advice about nutrition combined with an unfailing instinct for how to handle any situation where food is involved—life. It has seen me through a hectic schedule and travels all over the world, good times and not so good times. Heather understands the life of the busy Wall Street Person even if they don't work on Wall Street. She offers information everyone needs and deserves."*
> —JODY GOTTFRIED ARNHOLD, CHAIRMAN, BOARD OF DIRECTORS,
> BALLET HISPANICO

The Wall Street Commute

"*My commute takes me just over an hour each way. I've never really minded the time I spend on the train, but I know it's taken its toll. I just have almost no spare time. When you add the business dinners I have and the occasional travel, it's pretty obvious I don't have much time for myself. And my weight was really getting to be a problem, but frankly I couldn't imagine what I could do about it. I knew I couldn't follow a diet. My life is not regulated enough and my eating patterns certainly aren't. My doctor sent me to Heather because she said that if I didn't do something about the weight it would start to affect my health. Also, my clothes were all tight and I really just didn't feel good. Heather helped me figure out how to get on top of my eating. She made me realize that I'd been using my long work hours as an excuse to not be healthier, which is pretty crazy when you think about it. But I'm a new man now. Friends are asking me how I did it, and on my last trip to Hong Kong I got fitted for a batch of new suits. I've never felt better. I still don't think I exercise enough, but the fifteen pounds I've lost so far tell the story: at least I'm moving in the right direction.*"

—JOHN H., SPORTS AGENT

Here's the scenario: it's dark, it's cozy, you're deep in your Tuscan dream—drifting over sunny hill towns—when suddenly a fire truck siren drops you to earth. But it's not a fire truck: it's your alarm. It's 5:30 A.M., and it seems your head barely hit the pillow and it's time to get up and do it all over again. You're the Fred Astaire of the commuter shuffle and they're playing your tune.

I have clients who endure grueling commutes, week in and week out. They leap out of bed at gruesome hours. They grab something to eat on the way out the door—a piece of toast, a few mouthfuls of cereal—not because they're hungry but because it's an unconscious act, a habit rooted deep in their subconscious that they believe will help them wake up. They get to the train or bus or, if they're driving, a drive-through food window or deli, and grab something else. Maybe a big coffee drink and a Danish. Maybe a bagel. Something to make the long commute more pleasant. By the time they get to the office—sometimes almost three hours after rising—they're actually hungry. Now they're ready for some breakfast. So they think about maybe a ham and egg with cheese on a roll from the deli and another big coffee.

Before you know it, it's 10 A.M. and they've consumed over one thousand calories—for many people, more than half of their daily requirement. Worst of all, most of the calories were consumed unconsciously and without much satisfaction. Moreover, they're still facing lunch and dinner and perhaps a business drink date after work. These same people face a similar problem in reverse at the end of the day. It's no wonder commuters struggle with unique weight control issues.

Here are the three facts of commuter life that can make weight loss a challenge:

THE SYMPATHY SNACK. Face it: it's hard to commute. You feel frustrated because you spend so much time en route, away from your home and family and not even at work! You feel sorry for yourself because you're not where you want to be and you work really, really hard and . . . well . . . like they say in all the commercials these days, you deserve it. It's a pretty small compensation for the time you put in. Enter the sympathy snack: a giant whipped cream coffee drink, a scone, a buttered bagel . . . So you gain a little weight. What the heck. You've got no time for exercise anyhow and there's nothing you can do about your time on the road and you'll cope with it all someday in the future. When it comes to your weight and your health, you feel hopeless and trapped. Pass the doughnuts.

Does all that sound too familiar? If so, it's time to change your mindset. It's time to ditch the sympathy snack and get control of your commute. The brief satisfaction you feel munching a bagel on the train really doesn't make up for the dismay you feel at your ever-tighter waistband. Don't worry about exercise now. Put it out of your mind. It's true that you don't have time for it. But you *do* have time to strategize your commute so time on the train becomes productive or at least not destructive. I'm going to show you how to succeed at transforming your commute by eliminating the sympathy snacks so you won't even miss them.

THE COMMUTER SLUMP. You probably don't recognize it, but your blood sugar is enduring wild swings as a result of your commute-induced eating patterns. The highly refined carbs (think pastries, bagels, doughnuts) combined with caffeine that get you going in the morning give you immediate boosts of blood sugar. But they're inevitably followed by those grim slumps that leave you feeling wasted and desperate for another cup of coffee and a sympathy snack. You're locked in a pattern that affects not only your weight but also your general energy levels, to say nothing of your moods. It's not surprising that this yo-yoing of energy levels can affect your productivity at work as well as your ability to resist high-calorie food.

Many of my commuting clients complain of feeling tired all the time. They ascribe this to the toll that their travel time takes on them, but they are often, in fact, suffering from "sugar hangovers": they have trouble sleeping, they wake up tired, and they depend on sugary snacks and caffeine to keep them going. *These folks rarely make any connection between what they eat and their erratic energy levels.* They're amazed to find that once they start following the Wall Street Diet, their moods stabilize and their energy levels remain constant. I've had many clients tell me that they could get by on less sleep once they refined their eating habits the Wall Street way. In fact, I *don't* think they need less sleep— and I don't recommend that they try to get less than a healthy seven or eight hours—but I find it significant that many people report that a healthy eating pattern can boost energy levels throughout their day.

Eating the right types of foods—foods that boost your performance ability—is a cornerstone of the Wall Street Diet. The goal in the morning is to increase your body's synthesis of neurotransmitters. Neurotransmitters are chemicals that the brain uses to send messages among nerve cells. Certain neurotransmitters excite and others calm. Studies have shown that when your brain is producing the neurotransmitters dopamine and norepinephrine you feel more alert and focused. How do you stimulate the production of these chemicals? You eat protein foods. That's why it's important to have a protein food in the morning as you start your day. While refined carbs—sympathy snacks—may slow you down (and bounces in blood sugar exacerbate this effect), the protein foods I recommend for breakfast will have the opposite effect. When you substitute healthy snacks and a real breakfast for sympathy snacks, you'll begin to enjoy the sense of serenity and control—as well as the weight loss—that will serve you in your work as well as your weight loss efforts.

THE "X-OUT" EXERCISE SYNDROME. It's true. You really can't exercise. You don't have one minute to spare in your day. I'm an exercise enthusiast myself—as well as a health care professional—so I know how important exercise is, but I've worked with countless frazzled commuters who struggle with their weight and I feel their pain. For most of them, trying to squeeze forty-five minutes or even twenty minutes of daily exercise into their routine would be enough to put them over the edge. I can see it in their eyes when I meet with them and talk about their daily routines: "I'm warning you—if you ask me to exercise, I will go home and eat a Twinkie." So take a deep breath. Relax. I'm not going to push it now. But please pause and think about this as it could give you a fresh perspective on your struggle with weight: for many commuters the fact that they can't exercise allows them to adopt the position that they can't do *anything* about their weight and their health. The mantra is: "I have no time to eat well, no time to exercise, no time to lose weight. Maybe someday but not today." These people are smart and driven, and they tend to have an all-or-nothing attitude. So their rationale is, if they can't exercise—if they can't adopt a completely healthy lifestyle—there's no point in half measures. The demands of work and family make them feel trapped and hopeless. They give up.

I'll discuss exercise in detail in "The Wall Street Weekend" (page 186), but for now I want to tell you commuters something important. You won't need extra time to eat well the Wall Street way. You really won't. You don't have to beat yourself up about skipping the gym. You can and will lose weight and feel better. So don't let your crushing schedule and your inability to spend time exercising rule out a slimmer, healthier you.

SLEEP YOUR WAY SLIM *Recent research has shown that there's an intimate link between sleep habits and weight control. One study at Columbia University found a clear link between the risk of being obese and the number of hours you sleep each night, even after controlling for depression, physical activity, alcohol consumption, ethnicity, level of education, age, and gender. In this study, those who slept four hours or less per night were 73 percent more likely to be obese than those who slept seven to nine hours per night. Those sleeping five hours at night had a 50 percent higher risk and those who got six hours—a common sleep span for many of my clients—were still 23 percent more likely to be substantially overweight. A major key to this link seems to be the role played by the hormone leptin, which acts as an appetite suppressant.* A study on sleep and leptin found that people who slept less than five hours a night had a significant decrease in leptin as well as a significant increase in gherlin, a hormone that triggers hunger. So the decreased leptin and the increased gherlin seemed to act together to powerfully increase appetite. While I recognize that many people who commute, travel, and entertain for work find that their sleep time suffers, I still urge folks to do their best to establish and maintain good sleep habits.*

The Sympathy Snack, the Commuter Slump, and the X-Out Exercise work hand in hand to push you into a downward spiral that results in weight gain and a general feeling of hopelessness about your health and

---

* Gangwisch, J. E., Malaspina, D., Boden-Albala, B., Heymsfield, S. B. "Inadequate sleep as a risk factor for obesity: analyses of the NHANES I." *Sleep* 28(10) (October 1, 2005): 1289–96.

your excess pounds. But don't despair! You can lift yourself up. You can be successful. I've seen it happen countless times. You just need some inspiration and some specific techniques to help you manage the considerable stresses and time shortages that make healthy eating a challenge.

How to Manage Your Morning

You've probably heard that breakfast is the most important meal of the day. You picture a family sitting around the table, Dad reading the paper, Mom pouring the juice, and everyone enjoying their hot cereal and fresh fruit. You shrug your shoulders and think, "How quaint, but that's got nothing to do with me." Of course that's not *your* breakfast, and it never will be on most weekday mornings, but that's no reason to throw in the towel and grab a scone and coffee at the train station. You can create your own nutritious version of a healthy, low-cal, satisfying breakfast if you plan ahead and break free of your highly caffeinated, high-carb routine. Breakfast isn't brain surgery: it's simple. A protein and some fiber. I'll show you how.

Keep in mind that breakfast can be a moveable feast. You don't have to have a full breakfast at 6 or 7 A.M. or any particular time. The best time to eat breakfast is when you're *hungry* for it. Why? *Because calories consumed out of habit are wasted willpower*. Many people are not hungry early in the morning, but they eat out of habit or compulsion. Many people who grab something going out the door don't even enjoy what they're eating. If you're not hungry for the calories, don't eat them. This doesn't mean you should skip breakfast. It *really is* the most important meal of the day. For Wall Streeters, that means two things:

- Breakfast is the meal that research has shown is most important to weight loss. Those who eat breakfast are more successful at losing weight and at maintaining a healthy weight.

- Breakfast is the meal that you're best able to control. You usually eat it alone so there's no social pressure. You are usually in a good and optimistic frame of mind in the morning (A new day! I can do it!) and better able to make good choices.

Timing Your Breakfast

So you cannot skip breakfast. It's your out-of-the-starting-gate best opportunity to have a good diet day. But you have to make a decision about when to eat. For most people I suggest that they save breakfast until they get to work and then eat it in their office. Most people are not hungry when they get up and don't even begin to feel hungry until around 9 or 9:30 A.M. So have a mug of tea or coffee, black or with skim milk, before you leave the house if your schedule allows for this. If you do feel hungry, have a quick snack that's less than 60 calories. This snack could be

- a piece of fruit,

- a Fiber Rich cracker and 1 Laughing Cow Light wedge (or Laughing Cow Bite), or

- a Dannon 60-calorie Light & Fit yogurt or Light & Fit smoothie

Grab another tea or coffee at the train if you want to. Remember that even a skim latte has around two hundred calories, so you're really best off sticking with plain tea if possible. Just that simple switch from a higher-calorie coffee drink to tea can save lots of calories.

THINK AHEAD *Do you have a breakfast meeting in the office or at a restaurant? If so, it's definitely best to have only tea or coffee before you leave home or en route to work.*

Once you leave the house, you should work to shift the focus of your morning ride from food to something else—something positive. Some folks like to work their BlackBerrys. Others read the paper, make notes for work, scroll through family photos on their iPhone, or listen to their iPods. You can learn a language or listen to books on tape or even catch up on your sleep. I have a client who does isometric exercises on the train while she reads the paper.

If you can't eat your breakfast at the office for logistical reasons or because you really are hungry in the morning, then you do have to have something to eat before you leave the house. This may mean you'll need to get up a little earlier, but that shouldn't be too much of a challenge. You can prepare any number of things the night before and just eat them in the morning, either at home or on the train. The key for those who are eating before they get to work—either at home or on the train—is to limit themselves to *one* healthy breakfast. Once you're finished with your breakfast, you're finished. No coffee wagon at ten. No bagel from the place in the lobby. No frosted carbs from the tray in the office kitchen.

If you've saved your breakfast for work, try to eat as soon as you get there. You don't want your morning to get swallowed up by meetings and phone calls, so that you find yourself having skipped breakfast and facing lunchtime in a state of total, irrational starvation.

The Wall Street Diet Power Prescription Breakfasts

I think of breakfast as a prescription: you figure out what you need to take and you just do it every day. It's like brushing your teeth. It doesn't take a lot of thought or mental gymnastics. While lunch and dinner take certain strategic skills, breakfast should be a no-brainer. As I mentioned in The Plan, many people—Phase Eaters—have the same breakfast every day for weeks on end (and sometimes the same lunch) before shifting to another phase for weeks. While I think it's better to vary your breakfasts a bit, if you're more comfortable with a simple routine, stick with it.

The cornerstone of a power prescription breakfast is protein combined with enough fiber to hold you through the morning. Protein will help you concentrate at work and will give you the energy you need to get through a demanding morning.

Here are the Power Prescription Breakfasts:

CEREALS. Choose one with more than 5 grams of fiber, such as Kashi Go Lean, Heart to Heart, Fiber One, etc. You should serve yourself the portion size as listed on the box—usually one-half to three-quarters of a cup (see Shopping List, pages 305–06) with half a cup of low-fat, skim, or soy milk. (Clean Plate Club Eaters should choose cereal only if they can resist snacking on it later in the day and if they can limit themselves to *one* serving for breakfast.)

YOGURT. Zero to two percent plain Greek yogurt with a half cup of any approved cereal and one fruit. You can use any of the Shopping List (page 308) yogurts. If the yogurt is fruit-flavored, it counts as the fruit, so no additional fruit should be added. For the CPCers who can't have a bowl of cereal because of portion control issues, adding it to a yogurt works perfectly because the cereal addition is finite. (When traveling, you can crumble a Nature Valley granola bar—one-half for females and a whole bar for males—in place of the cereal.)

EGGS. Four-egg-white omelet or Egg Beaters, with Laughing Cow Light cheese or vegetables, plus two Fiber Rich crackers or wrapped in a La Tortilla wrap to create a breakfast wrap; or two hard-boiled eggs with two Fiber Rich crackers and one fruit.

OATMEAL. One cup cooked oatmeal. Choose McCann's, Arrowhead Mills (fruit-flavored or regular), Kashi Go Lean, or Quaker (nonflavored regular or weight-control). Many of these oatmeals come in instant packets, which are excellent for CPCers and also for in-office breakfasts. They can be quickly made in a coffee mug with boiling water. You can add one fruit (not dried fruit) to the oatmeal, plus, if desired, one tablespoon ground flaxseed or slivered almonds or one hard-boiled egg.

COTTAGE CHEESE. A half cup of cottage cheese with two Fiber Rich crackers and a fruit. Some men may find that they need up to a cup of cottage cheese, and they can choose 0 percent, 1 percent, or 2 percent fat. Clean Plate Clubbers do better with individual four-ounce packs of cottage cheese.

MORE, DIFFERENT COTTAGE CHEESE. Some of my clients have issues with the texture of cottage cheese. These folks love Friendship 1 percent whipped cottage cheese, which resembles cream cheese. Try it on a Fiber Rich cracker with some ground pepper and a tomato; with sugar-free jam; or with chopped chives.

PEANUT BUTTER. One and a half tablespoons of peanut butter with two Fiber Rich crackers and one teaspoon of jam or half a banana or any other fruit. (Most CPCers can't do peanut butter from a jar: they should stick to the Justin's packets, which are so nicely portion controlled.)

GRAB AND GO OPTIONS. *Bars:* Lärabar, Kashi TLC, Nature Valley granola bars, Luna Sunrise, or any bar on the Shopping List (page 311) that's not coated in chocolate. *Shakes:* Myoplex Light or Myoplex Carb Sense ready-to-drink shakes.

The Long and Hungry Road Home

For many people, the end-of-the-day commute is a major diet challenge. While breakfast, once you've figured it out, can be a prescription, the long and winding road home has physical and emotional obstacles that make it especially tough to stick to your goals. Earlier, we saw the hapless morning commuter, sleepily grabbing refined carbs and caffeine at every way station along the way. The same temptations confront you on your way home, but now you're tired. Your resistance is down. Maybe the day didn't work out as you'd hoped. In fact, maybe it was a pretty awful day. But even if the job went really well, you're still feeling the effects of those draining hours of work and you're tired. For some folks, the fatigue at the end of the day can have the effect of a cocktail: they lose their focus and some of their ability to make good decisions. And they're running a food gauntlet with drive-through temptations from the minute they leave the parking lot. Or else there's the hot pretzel at the station, the candy bar that leaped out at you when you bought your ticket . . . You're probably hungry and you're looking at a long stretch between your desk and home. And then maybe another stretch between kicking off your shoes and finally getting dinner.

Here's how to manage the evening commute:

- Have some hot tea at 3 or 4 P.M. if you can. It will fill you up a bit, calm you down, and help you face the challenges at the end of the day. If you're particularly sensitive to caffeine, be sure to drink an herb tea. Celestial Seasonings Sleepy Time has a nice flavor, and I promise it won't put you to sleep at your desk.

- Save your Fun Snack—your bar or soy crisps, for example—for the trip home. This will take the edge off your hunger and help hold you until dinner. If you're hungry in the afternoon, enjoy 2 Fiber Rich crackers with tea.

- A few of my commuting clients actually eat dinner on the way home if they have a long commute. This can be a turkey sandwich, for example. Once they get home, they have only a light snack before bed. This takes some preparation: most folks buy the sandwich at lunchtime so they're not slowed down on their way home. If this approach works for you, great. The negative to this technique is that it robs you of the pleasure of a truly relaxed meal at home—something most of us savor.

- Don't forget to drink your water in the afternoon. Staying hydrated will help to keep you full and also help fight fatigue.

- You may want to use some travel time to call home, if anyone is there, and strategize about dinner. Do you need to pick up a frozen dinner on the way home? Is someone at home ordering out? If so, you can request your favorite light dish.

Home at Last

You take a deep breath and close the door behind you. You're exhausted. Maybe there are still plates of food around from what your family ate. Maybe the kitchen is clean and silent. In either case, you have to manage your evening meal so you don't fall back on that Wall Streeter trap, the dreaded Mishmash Dinner.

The Mishmash Dinner is famous among my clients, many of whom are connoisseurs of Mishmash eating. Here's how you find yourself on the slippery slope of the Mishmash Dinner. You get home, exhausted and starving. You grab two chicken nuggets from the plate on the table and swipe them in a pool of ketchup. Then you decide that, because there's nothing healthy at hand, and/or because you have no time or interest in cooking anything, you're going to just have a bowl of nutritious cereal with some skim or soy milk. So you do. And then you have another because it's healthy, after all, and how many calories can it have? And then just one more shake of cereal to use up the milk. And then you get changed and settle in to watch some TV, but you're still hungry because you haven't had a real dinner, and that can't be fair, so you have another handful of cereal and a couple of sticks of string cheese and a few crackers. Then you notice that there are still some cookies in that box over there so you grab a couple. And now you begin to feel that the evening is a lost cause, and you'll just try again tomorrow, so you break out the chips and have a few spoonfuls of frozen cookie dough. The lyrics to the Mishmash theme song go something like "I'm sure I'll get much slimmer 'cause I didn't eat my dinner. I won't count this little bit . . ." By the time you fall into bed, you've consumed sufficient calories for an entire day in the few hours you've been home, and you've prepped yourself to wake up with a sugar/carb hangover.

How do you avoid the Mishmash Dinner? You know the answer. You probably heard it from your mother years ago: eat dinner like a normal person! Here are some strategies to get you back on track with a healthy dinner following a long commute:

- **CHANGE BEFORE YOU ENTER THE KITCHEN.** Don't come in the door and rush right into the kitchen. You're tired and hungry and you're too likely to slide into a Mishmash Dinner. Get out of your work clothes. Wash your face and hands. The simple act of getting changed out of your work clothes and creating a transition from work to home life sets the stage for a real dinner, one that is a satisfying ritual.

■ **STOCK SOME HEALTHY FROZEN DINNERS.** I have many
clients who tell me that, well, they thought about frozen dinners, but aren't they high in sodium? And aren't they too high in
calories? These are often the same people who then habitually
consume Mishmash Dinners with sodium and calorie counts up
in the stratosphere! You can find healthy frozen dinners that are
excellent alternatives to a fresh home-cooked meal. While I
wouldn't recommend that you eat them every evening, they're a
tasty and satisfying choice for those nights when the most you
can do is peel back a lid and hit some numbers on the microwave. Here's a big benefit of a frozen dinner: it's finite. Once it's
gone, it's gone. You can't have second helpings. Eating an occasional frozen dinner—a low-calorie, healthy frozen dinner—can
help reinforce the idea of portion control. It shows you what
300 or 350 calories really looks like. It also shows you how you
should feel after a meal: not stuffed but just pleasantly satisfied.
You go to bed full, but you wake up with a good hunger because
you've eaten an appropriate—rather than a linebacker—dinner
the night before. See the Wall Street Shopping List (pages
313–14) for top frozen dinner picks.

■ No time to shop? Consider using a supermarket delivery service to keep healthy, prepared dinners stocked in your fridge.
(See page 38 for some delivery service options.)

■ If there's someone at home—a partner or an older child—ask
that person to fix a plate for you. Most people are more than
willing to do this to help you stick to your weight loss goals.
Pulling a lovely plate of chicken and salad, say, out of the fridge
is both emotionally and physically satisfying.

FACE UP TO FROZEN PASTA! *I have many clients who have been on
low-carb diets and are terrified of pasta. But sometimes a frozen low-cal
lasagna or stuffed shell dinner can make an excellent, satisfying choice. If
you have a craving for pasta, indulge it with a healthy option. It may keep
you from losing control with a boatload of fettucine Alfredo in a fancy Italian restaurant.*

How to Stop Night Eating

You changed clothes. You ate. You have a little time before bed. So you're thinking, well, maybe just a few crackers or a spoonful of Rocky Road while you watch the news . . . Late-night eating is a serious challenge for countless people, especially Clean Plate Club Eaters. It's comforting, it's habit-forming. Many of my clients struggle with late-night eating, and it's easy to see why. Like alcohol, mindless eating can be soothing. You're wound up all day and you run from meeting to meeting and phone call to phone call, always stressed and always performing. You eat during the day, but oftentimes you're so distracted you don't even taste your food. You are so in control in the course of the day that when you get home, your psyche is screaming for release. You want to put on a pair of sweat-pants, grab a bowl of popcorn, and let it all wash away. This routine evening eating can be a hard habit to break. But break it you must or you'll demolish all the positive steps you've taken during the day to eat light, healthy meals and move closer to your weight loss goals. The trick is to find alternative activities—a way to redirect your energies—that will satisfy your need to relax and feel comforted.

Consider these tips to help you conquer the late-night munchies:

- If you're a Controlled Eater, you can have one sweet treat with dinner. You should keep it to under 80 calories. This could be a piece of fruit, a Dannon Light & Fit Yogurt (frozen, so it takes a long time to eat!), a sugar-free chocolate pudding, etc. (See Wall Street Shopping List, page 312, for suggestions of snacks for Controlled Eaters.) Eat your sweet immediately after dinner, as a dessert. This satisfies your sweet tooth, but it eliminates thoughts like "Well, I'll save it for later and maybe have two of them or maybe something else as long as I'm in the kitchen."

- Know yourself. If late-night eating is a problem for you, try to eliminate the foods that you tend to snack on. If you're a Clean Plate Club Eater (and assuming that others in your household don't need them), you might have to get rid of pickable, poppable, dippable, unstoppable foods like cereals, chips, pretzels, cookies, etc. If you can't eliminate these snacks, keep them in a cabinet that's off-limits to you.

- Are you eating mindlessly or are you really hungry? If you're really hungry and feel you need to eat something, go for the Turkey Solution. This is why you've got those quarter-pound bags of sliced turkey in the fridge. Eat one bag of turkey. This will satisfy any real hunger you experience, but it's highly unlikely to set off a binge. By the way, don't put the turkey on a piece of bread or a Fiber Rich cracker, or dab it with mayo or mustard: this snack is meant to be eaten plain and unadorned.

- The kitchen is closed! When you're finished eating dinner, you're finished in the kitchen. Make it a point to avoid kitchen reentry after your evening meal. This is especially important for Clean Plate Club Eaters.

- Take a shower. It's relaxing and cleansing. It washes off your day. When you feel clean and refreshed, you're less likely to nibble. Most people find that after a shower they feel strengthened and less likely to succumb to mindless snacking.

- Do personal maintenance. Do your nails. Check your wardrobe. Pay your bills. These routine activities keep you out of the kitchen and can break the TV/snack habit.

- Brush your teeth. (And floss for a change!) Most people aren't eager to eat once they've brushed their teeth.

- Use whitening strips on your teeth. They prevent you from eating for about thirty minutes.

- Find a distraction. Read. Play Sudoku. Take up knitting or needlework. Download some music from iTunes. Exercise DVDs can be a good way to unwind (see page 199 for suggestions).

- Controlled Eaters can have an evening beverage: try an herb tea. Chamomile tea is a good nighttime choice. Or try a low-cal cocoa: mix 1 teaspoon of Ghirardelli cocoa mix in warm skim milk. It's only about forty calories and is filling and calming. Swiss Miss has a sugar-free hot chocolate with only twenty-five calories a serving.

- Create a ritual. One of my clients sits in the bedroom with her husband at night and they each enjoy one glass of wine. They catch up on their day and relax. This is the opposite of mindless eating: it's a pleasurable ritual. It won't work for everyone, but if you have a partner and you're looking for a way to relax at night, it's a good option.

The Wall Street Commuting Cheat Sheets

Some deli breakfast choices:

- 1 cup 1% cottage cheese, small fruit salad (optional: add 2 Fiber Rich crackers)

- 4 egg whites with 1 slice of cheese on a plate, small fruit salad (request low or no oil to cook the eggs)

- 4 egg whites on 2 pieces of wheat toast, 1 slice of cheese, 1 piece of fruit (counts as Juicy Carb)

- 2 hard-boiled eggs, small fruit salad (optional: add 2 Fiber Rich crackers)

- Nonfat yogurt, small fruit salad (or light smoothie— Dannon/Stonyfield Farm)

- Peanut butter on wheat toast with ½ banana (tell them very light on the pb) (counts as Juicy Carb)

Some at-home breakfasts:
(Can do any of the breakfasts above at home plus these.)

- Cereal choice from Shopping List, pages 305–6. Stick to serving on box and have with ½ cup low fat or soy milk plus 1 fruit, cut up

- 1.5 tablespoon peanut butter with Thomas' Light Wheat English Muffin with 1 teaspoon jam or ½ banana or with 2 Fiber Rich crackers

- 0–2% Greek Yogurt with ½ cup cereal and 1 cup berries

- ¼ cup steel-cut oatmeal (make night before and reheat), makes about 1 cup cooked; add 1 cup fruit (can add 1 tablespoon ground flaxseeds, slivered almonds, or 1 hard-boiled egg to make it more filling)

- 2 MorningStar Veggie Links, 2 crackers, and 1 fruit or 2 Al Fresco/Casual Gourmet chicken sausages with 2 crackers and/or fruit

- Smoothie/shake: easiest is Myoplex Light package with 10 ice cubes, and you can add 1 tablespoon instant coffee or 1 packet Swiss Miss sugar-free cocoa mix, and/or ½ cup skim milk. Or you can just take 1 cup frozen berries with 8 ounces skim milk or yogurt and ice and add 1 tablespoon ground flaxseed and / or 1 tablespoon peanut butter or 1 scoop Designer Whey Protein.

Some breakfast choices for fancy restaurants:

- 2 poached eggs with sliced tomatoes and 1 slice wheat toast

- Egg-white veggie (load up on mushrooms, spinach, peppers, onions, tomatoes) omelet with 1 slice of cheese, lettuce, tomato, and 1 slice toast optional (Virgin Dieter can add 2 slices Canadian bacon if still hungry and skip toast)

- Eggs Florentine, extra spinach, no muffin, no sauce

- Eggs Benedict, muffin equals Juicy Carb, no hollandaise sauce

- Oatmeal (request it to be made with water or skim milk), no sugar, cinnamon OK and fruit OK

- Some restaurants, even the fancy ones, will have fiber cereal; you can have a bowl with skim milk and a small fruit salad on the side.

Some breakfasts to keep in your office:

- Justin's peanut butter packet (classic peanut), plus 2 Fiber Rich crackers and fruit (½ banana)

- 1 packet oatmeal (Arrowhead Mills makes a good fruit-flavored organic oatmeal) plus fruit

- Keep box of cereal in office and add ½ cup to a light/nonfat yogurt. Enjoy with piece of fruit (for Controlled Eaters only)

- Breakstone's snack-sized 2% cottage cheese; have it with 2 crackers and a fruit

- Put cereal in a mug and add skim milk

- Myoplex Light ready to drink

- Bar breakfast: Lärabar, Kashi TLC crunch bar, Luna Sunrise (look for bar under 200 calories that does not have a chocolate coating) and add a fruit if needed

Some breakfast nightmares (with calories):

AT DELI
- Muffin (400–600)

- Scone (490–650)

- Yogurt parfait (500–600)

- Bagel (400 without topping)

AT RESTAURANTS
- Einstein Brothers Santa Fe Bagel Omelet Sandwich (720)

- IHOP Colorado Omelet meal (1220/83 grams fat)

- Carl's Jr. Low-carb Breakfast Bowl (900)

- IHOP Classic Combo Country-Fried Steak/Eggs (1531)

- Jamba Juice Peanut Butter Moo'd (840)

The Wall Street Weekend: Eating Well at Home and High-dividend Exercise Tips

"It's no longer hard for me to eat carefully during the week. I'm on the go all the time with work, and my schedule is quite regulated. I've learned to make good choices at lunches and business dinners. But the weekend was another story. I used to be out of control. It was like I was let out of a corral to forage in the wild! It usually started with Friday night, when I felt such a sense of pleasure that the work week was over that it really seemed like I deserved to celebrate. When I got home, I felt entitled to pull on some sweatpants and relax. The biggest issue was that I could never figure out how to deal with being surrounded by food all day at home. Heather changed all that. Now being at home isn't a signal to lose control. My weekends definitely take a little more thought than my weekdays, but I'm managing them well and I'm finding that Monday morning no longer means a 'food hangover.' I've lost twenty-three pounds so far and I'm still losing."

LAURA Z., ANALYST, INTERNATIONAL BANK

Ah yes . . . Weekends, vacations, retirement. They're downtime, relax time, hang loose time. . . . And that's the problem! There's nothing a hard worker enjoys more than a well-deserved break, even if some of it is spent on the BlackBerry. At least you're home, enjoying family and friends, sleeping late, and recharging. The trick, for those trying to lose weight, is to embrace the relaxed ambience of time away from the office while maintaining some control over your food intake. The goal I present to my clients is this: try to be thinner on Monday than you were on Friday. If you can't tighten your belt on Monday morning, at least promise yourself on Friday morning that you won't be loosening it when the new workweek rolls around in a couple of days. It's easier to maintain control over food intake when you have a structure. The ideas suggested in this chapter are all about creating your own personal eating structure on the weekends (and vacations and other at-home times) so you can reach your thinner-on-Monday goal.

The Friday Challenge

Your Friday sets the tone for the weekend, and your goal for the day is to keep it clean! Friday can be a tough day. It's the end of the week. You're exhausted. The stress has accumulated and your resistance is down. And most of the people in the office are moving into party mode. The slippery slope can begin with office pizza and goes quickly downhill from there. You meet friends for drinks that become more drinks and a late-night food binge, or you head home, where the family has ordered in greasy Chinese food. You wind up the workweek standing in front of the fridge at midnight, finishing off a pint of ice cream. It's very hard to wake up on Saturday morning and feel refreshed and positive when you are suffering from a sugar and/or alcohol hangover. In this state of mind, the weekend can already seem a loss.

The solution? Hold things together on Friday. Start the day strong with a good, healthy breakfast. Keep the eating clean all day so your reserves of willpower will be there when you need them at night. Skip any office pizza. Pick a clean lunch—a salad and protein combo is a great choice. Hold off on your afternoon snack until late in the day so that you'll find either after-work drinks or the family dinner less tempting. If you're meeting friends for drinks, just decide to order food, too. That way you'll avoid a late-night unhealthy binge. Get a chicken Caesar and go light on the dressing, or have a burger and skip the bun. If you're headed home to the family, call ahead and check on dinner. If they're ordering in, request your favorite steamed dish. When you hold your Fridays together, the rest of the weekend is less of a challenge and you really will be able to tighten your belt on Monday morning.

Start Your Saturday Strong

For most people, breakfast sets the tone for the day. And on a Saturday morning, that can actually mean for the next day as well. Many clients report that a Saturday morning pancake binge with the kids used to ruin their entire weekend in terms of food choices. The mountain of pancakes, swimming in syrup, seemed to ease the skids into a fatty lunch, endless snacks, and a calorie-is-king dinner. The key is to start off on the right foot. You don't know what the day will bring, but if you have a healthy breakfast, you're on your way to a successful weekend. I know that this isn't always easy if you're accustomed to large family breakfasts or leisurely brunches in the neighborhood, but you can do it! Make the decision to begin your weekend with a healthy, light Wall Street breakfast. You can still make pancakes for the kids; just make sure to have your own breakfast—cereal, yogurt, an egg-white omelet—on hand for you to enjoy while the kids chow down. Of course this means planning ahead to be sure that your breakfast ingredients are available, but most people will find that they're eating the same breakfast that they eat on weekdays, so the kitchen should already be stocked appropriately. If you're eating out, check the Wall Street Cheat Sheets for healthy breakfast restaurant choices (page 256).

CHECK YOUR CALORIE FORECAST. It's always important to look ahead to your day and assess what you'll be eating and when, but it's especially critical on the weekends. Once you're free of your weekday routine, mealtimes can shift, fast-food restaurants can become part of the parenting landscape, and treats like brunches and restaurant dinners can pop up. Of course you should enjoy these mealtime events—they're part of the pleasure of downtime—but you should figure them into your daily calorie intake. For example, if you know that you're going to have a leisurely dinner with friends at a new restaurant that you're looking forward to trying, then plan on a light lunch and a satisfying afternoon snack. If, on the other hand, dinner is going to be a pickup meal of leftovers and a movie at home, you might want to take that opportunity to make lunch a more substantial meal.

START THE CLOCK WITH YOUR FIRST MEAL. When you're used to leaping out of bed at 5:30 A.M., it can be pure bliss to snooze until 11 A.M. If that's your pleasure, then enjoy! But don't roll out of bed at eleven, eat breakfast, and segue right into lunch an hour or two later. Start your day with the meal you get up for, which for most late sleepers means that they'll begin the day with lunch. So if you get up at eleven, make lunch at noon your first meal and go on from there. (I promise you won't experience painful hunger pangs from skipping one meal!) If you do notice that you're especially hungry late in the afternoon, have a healthy snack.

FIRST, CONSIDER YOUR DINNER. Many people enjoy special dinners on the weekends—wheather at home, at friends' homes, or at restaurants. I advise clients to plan their day with their dinner in mind. Are you going out for a special meal? Are you having a dinner party at home? If you expect to eat a special meal at night, plan for it right from the beginning of the day with a light breakfast and lunch, and some well-planned snacks. Then you'll arrive at your dinner with a nice low-calorie balance for the day, but your snacks will prevent a ravenous blowout. You'll be able to enjoy your meal without straying into the diet danger zone. If you're a Clean Plate Clubber, it's usually best to plan for a later dinner.

FIGURE YOUR FAST FOOD. If you have kids, your weekends can be a blur of hockey practice, dance lessons, soccer games, and living in the car. And yes, fast food happens. So be prepared. You *can* eat fast food; you just have to order judiciously. See the Wall Street Cheat Sheets, High-dividend Chain Choices (page 237) for suggestions on the best fast-food picks at various restaurants. Sometimes fast-food meals will surprise you. At McDonald's, for example, the plain burger is 250 calories while the

Asian Salad with Crispy Chicken and dressing is 460 calories. At Burger King the burger is 290 calories and one packet of the honey mustard dressing is 270 calories! Obviously, you're better off having a plain burger than a salad with that high-cal dressing. A little education will help you avoid fast-food pitfalls and will allow you to enjoy a meal with the kids and keep hunger at bay. You may be surprised to see the low-cal, healthy options that most fast-food and chain restaurants have added to their menus.

FRIDAY NIGHT, NOT-SO-LIGHT *I caution clients that weighing themselves on a Saturday or a Sunday morning can be a mistake. I've heard too many tales of woe from clients who indulged in salty foods on Friday (at a Japanese restaurant or bar happy hour) and were horrified to see the number on the scale on Saturday morning, which reflected all the water they were retaining. Bloat is never fun, but when it rears its ugly head on a weekend, some people are propelled into a "lost weekend" of devil-may-care eating that takes a major toll on diet progress. If you might be discouraged by a small uptick on the scale, save your weigh-ins for weekdays, when you will find your busy schedule will better help you control your eating.*

MANAGE SNACKS. Snacks constitute a clear and present danger when you spend time at home. Clean Plate Clubbers, in particular, often struggle with time on their hands and all the food that's available to them in their own kitchens. The solution? You need a snack plan. You can slot in your afternoon Fun Snack, but many people find that on weekends they need filler snacks. The key strategy is to have a plethora of healthy snacks on hand and plan to eat them when they'll do you the most good. So, say at 2 P.M., you could have a fruit, and then an hour and a half later, enjoy your protein bar. At 5 P.M. you might have some cut-up pepper and cucumber, and then an hour later, munch on six almonds. Yes, this is more calories than you'd normally consume, but it will keep you satisfied, keep your blood sugar up, and it's ten times better than ripping open a bag of Doritos. So plan your snacks to keep you busy and full. Clean Plate Clubbers should always make a point of having their quarter-pound bags of sliced turkey on hand for the weekends. If they find that the cut vegetables, Fiber Rich crackers, fruit, etc., aren't satisfying them, they can settle down with a bag or two of sliced turkey.

Here's a safe snacking plan for both Controlled and Clean Plate Club Eaters. This chart reflects the maximum number of allowed snacks. It's a mental safety net to know you can have that much. But if you want to skip an item or two, that's fine.*

Snacking Plan

	FOR CONTROLLED EATERS	FOR CLEAN PLATE CLUB EATERS
2 P.M.	1 fruit	1 hand fruit
3:30 P.M.	bar or soy crisps	cut-up cucumber or pepper (or both)
5 P.M.	6 almonds	¼ pound turkey
6:30 P.M.	1 Fiber Rich with Laughing Cow	2 Fiber Rich
7 P.M.	2 5.5-ounce cans of low-sodium V8 with lemon over ice, or 1 packet of sugar-free hot chocolate or herbal tea	2 5.5-ounce cans of low-sodium V8 with lemon over ice, or 1 packet of sugar-free hot chocolate or herbal tea

A GREAT DIP FOR RELAXING WEEKENDS OR ENTERTAINING ANY TIME *Take a 0 or 2% Greek Yogurt and add in two tablespoons of Knorr veggie or onion soup mix and enjoy with cut-up celery, peppers, or cucumbers. This is good for both Clean Plate Club and Controlled Eaters. The sodium level is somewhat high, however, so those who are salt-sensitive should beware.*

STEP AWAY FROM THE PIZZA CRUST. If you're a parent at home with kids on weekends, you're probably preparing lots of food. Kids eat more

* If you eat every single snack, it adds up to only about 300 to 350 calories, which is far better than a bag of Doritos and a "Might-as-Well" weekend.

frequently than adults, and they're not interested, nor should we expect them to be, in "diet" food. It may be tough for you to throw out the kids' quarter of a sandwich, half a cookie, and innocent-looking wedge of pizza. But remember, those little bits and dabs of food take a real toll on your daily calorie intake. In fact, I've had a number of clients mystified by why they're not losing more weight when their meals are so healthy and low in calories. But when they carefully record their weekend (and sometimes weeknight) intake from their kids' plates, including French fries from their Happy Meals and other food that they couldn't bear to "waste," they saw in black and white why the scale wouldn't budge. If it helps to chew gum* or sip herb tea or hot water with lemon while cooking for your kids or cleaning up after their meals, do so. Some clients tell me that this trick saves them many calories. Sometimes it's just a question of being firm with yourself and looking forward to your own meals: do you really want to fill up on McDonald's fries when you're going to have a lovely dinner with your partner that evening? Wouldn't you rather splurge later on an extra glass of wine or a spoonful of dessert? One client had a terrific solution to her bad habit of postprandial plate surfing: as soon as her children were able, she taught them to clear their own plates, scrape them, and put them in the dishwasher.

AVOID THE "LOST SUNDAY." Sunday can present its own special challenges. It's usually a relaxed day. And clients often tell me that "relaxed" can sometimes spill over into "sloppy." If you have kids, they're doing homework or hanging around. You're reading the paper and taking it easy. Or maybe you had a late night out with too many martinis and then you find yourself at a brunch spot with friends and the bloody mary or mimosa comes with the meal and the bread basket is just too tempting and they have wild blueberry pancakes on the menu! It can be tempting to just "lose" the day and indulge in snacks and a Chinese take-out dinner. Try to plan your day so you'll avoid these pitfalls. A great solution if you wake up with a food or drink hangover is to get in a quick run or sweat at the gym, even if you do so just a half hour before your brunch date. You'll feel more energized and in control. You can always get in another gym session later

* If you're a CPCer, keep gum intake to under five sticks a day. Gum can cause a poppable, pickable bellyache.

if you have time, or do an active outing with the family. If you enjoy cooking, perhaps you'd like to make a healthy soup to enjoy during the week.

KEEP BUSY. There's perhaps no bigger challenge for a dieter than a rainy, quiet day at home, whether it's on a weekend, vacation, or even during a stretch between jobs or in retirement. The kitchen beckons and it's perfect weather for a carb festival. The solution is to plan ahead. My clients are goal-oriented, and they do well when they keep a to-do list for the weekend. It might include things like writing thank-you notes, buying a gift, cleaning out the closet, or scheduling exercise. These kinds of constructive, productive activities are satisfying, and even though they have nothing to do with food or dieting, accomplishing anything you set out to do strengthens resolve. The very best diversion? Physical exercise. A session at the gym can do wonders for your resolve. But if that doesn't suit you, a walk with a friend, a game of tennis, or a bike ride could be just what you need to burn a few calories, banish hunger, and boost resolve. It's very satisfying to settle in on Sunday night, after enjoying an active, busy, productive weekend. It makes Monday a much better day.

Some Food-free Weekend Suggestions

Download new DVDs to your iPod for your next trip

Download photos to your new iPhone

Use *www.Picasa.com* to organize digital photos

Clean off the desktop on your computer

Open that huge pile of mail

Buy and assemble a new piece of technology

Pay your bills

Clean out the closet and drop off clothes to Goodwill

Visit a grandparent

Get your car washed, or even better, detail your own car

After you food shop, prepare 1 to 2 meals for the week that you can freeze

---

What About Exercise?
The Wall Street Guide to Moving and Shaking

Here's my approach to exercise: when they come to see me, most clients are so overscheduled and busy that it would be counterproductive to insist that they work exercise into their schedules. It would simply cause more stress and might ultimately deter them from taking any steps at all to lose weight and improve their health. For many people, nonnegotiable exercise requirements can be the escape clause that super-busy people unconsciously seek. It goes something like this: you can't imagine that you could find time to exercise, and you don't much feel like doing it anyhow, so you figure it's not worth dieting either. Pass the scone. This is where, in my experience, strict adherence to exercise guidelines and timelines, valid as they may be, can lead us astray.

So how important is exercise? And what if you don't think you're going to be quick to jump on the treadmill no matter what the experts tell you? Well, it's one of the questions that has perplexed mankind from time immemorial. Along with which came first, the chicken or the egg, we struggle with what matters more if you want to lose weight, diet or exercise? Leaving the first question to the poultry people, we'll take a stab at the second. The bottom line is that in order to lose weight, you must burn more calories than you take in. It's simple math. There are two ways to achieve weight loss: eat fewer calories or burn extra calories by adding more physical activity to your routine. A combination of both diet *and* exercise seems to be the best prescription for effective long-term weight loss. On the other hand, there is convincing evidence that if you had to choose one single path—diet or exercise—diet alone is the more effective road to immediate weight loss. Many studies have compared results from reducing calories versus increasing exercise in terms of weight loss. In general, programs that focus on dietary change produce greater weight loss than programs that rely on exercise. Probably this is because research demonstrates that simple strategies like the ones in the Wall Street Diet—eliminating Dry Carbs, choosing carefully from restaurant menus, and managing alcohol and portion size—can quickly eliminate up to, say, 500 calories daily, while burning an extra

500 calories a day can be a much more difficult and time-consuming undertaking. So my position, particularly for my unique, busy, stressed-out clientele is: *start with your diet.*

This approach has proven to be effective time and again. Many of the people who come to see me have in fact avoided dealing with weight loss and their overall health because they've felt certain that they'd be instructed to exercise and they were convinced that they couldn't squeeze one more thing into their already overburdened days. Indeed, many clients tell me that when they see some of the popular "healthy living" recommendations—no alcohol, no coffee, an hour of daily exercise most days—they simply feel it's hopeless. In fact, I've been told by more than one client that they haven't bothered trying to improve their diets because they know they can't exercise so what's the point? This is unfortunate and also untrue. I can assure you that I've had countless clients who came to see me insisting that they couldn't exercise, who nonetheless became very successful at reaching their weight loss goals. Most of these people eventually began to exercise; some did not. But they all lost weight and gained health.

My time-tested reasons for making diet a primary focus are psychological. You don't exercise when you're told you must do it; you exercise when you already feel good and optimistic about your body. When you are overweight, you have a host of reasons not to exercise. For one thing, most of the people at the gym are already in great shape! This is the discouraging fact that sends too many people from the step class right to the bakery. For another, when you're not eating well, you don't feel good about your body. Your clothes are tight and you don't like the way you look in the mirror. (Gyms, of course, are filled with mirrors!) The last thing a discouraged, overburdened, overweight person wants to do is put on some spandex and stand in front of a mirror with a host of trim, toned gym rats.

Stress is another significant deterrent to exercise among my clientele. When you feel overworked, exhausted, and pulled in all directions by family obligations, you lose something of yourself. You not only feel uncomfortable in your clothes, but also a bit cranky, pressured, trying to serve everyone but you. Who wouldn't feel a little out of control under these circumstances and, to some degree, hopeless? But here's the good news: there is one thing you can control and that's what you eat. Whether you're on the road, rushing to a meeting, or heading home for family time, the one thing that you can say yes or no to is what you'll eat. So many aspects of your day are beyond your control. But what you choose to eat is not. When you appreciate that concept, it immediately takes your stress down a notch. It's both calming and empowering to recognize that food choices are totally up to you. Whatever else happens in your day, if you can say that at least you ate well, or at least you feel good about what you ate, that's a giant step in the right direction. For all these reasons, and because for most people eating well is easier to manage than exercising, I focus on diet first and foremost.

In the spirit of full disclosure, I should mention that exercise is an important part of my own life. I grew up with two parents who are marathon runners and exercise is as routine to me as brushing my teeth. Some of the people who come to see me are already avid exercisers. Some have personal trainers and work out regularly. Some are sporadic exercisers. If you already exercise, terrific! You're going to lose weight and reach your goals more quickly. But if you don't already exercise, don't worry. You'll get there on your own schedule.

Exercise 101

If exercise is something that's been on your back burner for so long that it's nothing but a charred crust of a good intention, don't despair. You're simply going to start with the food. I want all your energy and attention focused on what you eat. You're going to follow the Wall Street Diet for two weeks, or until your belt is one notch tighter. I promise you that when you reach that point, you'll be ready to move and shake.

Consider Julie's story. Julie is a risk manager at Morgan Stanley. She had recently been promoted and came to see me at a friend's recommendation because her promotion meant a higher profile at work and more entertaining. She had about thirty pounds to lose, and she wanted to look her best as she met new business contacts. She'd also realized that it was time to upgrade her wardrobe, and she didn't want to take that step until she got closer to her ideal weight. Julie hadn't exercised since high school and clearly wasn't interested in trying to start an exercise program. When I told her she shouldn't think about exercise at this point, I could see her whole body relax. Julie did extremely well on the diet. On her second visit she showed me menu printouts from all the restaurants she was now favoring. She'd selected the best choices on each. She had already lost four pounds. After one month, Julie had lost twelve pounds. By the time she came for her fourth visit, she looked terrific. I wasn't surprised when she told me she'd just started to exercise. She had joined a gym and was trying to get there in the morning twice a week and once on the weekend.

Julie is typical of countless clients who find that once they begin to lose weight, their outlook on exercise changes. As energy levels increase and clothes loosen and enthusiasm and confidence builds, exercise becomes a welcome activity rather than a burden. It's not that people suddenly find holes in their schedule that never existed before; it's more that they feel so good about the way they look that they want to amplify the good results they're getting. Exercise is definitely the best way to ramp up the benefits of a healthy, low-calorie diet. If I have two clients who are losing weight, the loss is almost invariably more apparent on the one who exercises. Exercise creates more muscle—more lean body mass—and this makes the body look trimmer. That's because exercise helps cut inches. It also increases motivation, and this is a critical factor in long-term success. Taking the time to exercise—scheduling it into your day—reinforces the idea that your health, and your weight, are priorities. You deserve to take the time required to exercise.

If you can't do it right off the bat, that's okay; relax. The day will come when you'll want to exercise. I promise!

My treatment of exercise here is not meant to be exhaustive. I simply want to convey the two critical points: you don't need to begin to exercise when you begin the diet (although if you're already exercising, continue and that will speed your progress). You can postpone it until your body tells you that the time is right. And second, when you do begin to exercise, you'll see and feel the difference. You can find a wealth of good information on exercise and different types of exercise. You can join a gym or simply walk with a friend. You can begin with a personal trainer or you can borrow a few good exercise books or tapes or CDs from the library and get started. Any steps you take to get more active will pay dividends in both the short and long term when it comes to your weight and your health.

Now I'd like to share some exercise pointers that you'll find useful:

- Exercise in the morning. Let's face it: almost all of us are just too tired after a day of work and too distracted by other activities and family to exercise at night. Early morning exercise boosts your metabolism all day. And think about it: what's twenty minutes out of your day? Especially when you spend that much time hitting the snooze button anyhow! Getting up early and exercising before your colleagues have opened their eyes makes you feel you're ahead of the game. No matter what your day holds, you'll feel good about taking care of yourself right at the start.

- Yes, it can be a struggle to get up early, especially if it's cold and dark. Try leaving your blinds open to allow whatever light there is into your bedroom in the morning. You may want to think about investing in a coffeemaker with a programmable clock so you can wake to the aroma of hot coffee (or tea: just put a few tea bags in the bottom of the carafe and use an empty filter).

- Log your exercise on your food diary. It helps to see what you've accomplished even if it's just a brisk walk around the block at lunchtime.

- A good basic exercise regime for beginners is to start with one twenty-minute session of cardiovascular-boosting activity two to three days a week. That might include walking, bicycling, elliptical . . . whatever activity suits you and that you enjoy. (You definitely are not going to be able to continue with any activity that you don't enjoy!) Hopefully you'll work up a sweat, because sweating is important. It feels good to sweat when you're stressed. It relaxes you and invigorates you at the same time. So I recommend that beginners focus on cardio first and only then consider weight training.

- Tapes and DVDs are great for busy people who want to exercise at home and when they travel without going to a gym. Leslie Sansone, for example, has some excellent walking programs on CDs that you can do at home or on the road. There's also a Yoga Zone Power Yoga for Strength and Endurance DVD that's a good choice for people who travel. It's set up as a 50-minute session that can be used on your laptop. It's very calming to do this at night, especially after a long, hard day of work. Because it's power yoga, it increases your heart rate while it strengthens you and helps promote flexibility. You might also look for a CD called *Fluidity* (*www.fluidity.com*). This mixes yoga, Pilates, and ballet and uses your body's weight for resistance so you engage all of your muscles.

- Check out your cable TV exercise offerings. Many cable services offer exercise-on-demand sessions that can be quite brief if you're pressed for time. Time Warner Cable in New York offers Exercise TV on demand, and their workouts run from five to thirty-eight minutes.

- If you are traveling, take the opportunity to turn your business trip into a spa trip. I've already talked about this in the chapter on business travel (pages 160–65). It's an excellent technique for boosting your weight loss over the course of a trip. You'll come home refreshed, energized, trimmer, and closer to your goal. Map out any time you might have for exercise before you leave on your trip and schedule it into your BlackBerry. Even if the hotel gym has only an exercise bike from 1965, get on it and do your twenty minutes.

- Use the Twenty-Minute Rule. I always tell my clients, just do it for twenty minutes. Whether it's walking or riding the exercise bike or doing basic exercises from an exercise tape, if you set a goal of twenty minutes, you'll most often find that you go longer. One client told me that she always set out to walk at lunch for twenty minutes and she never walked less than thirty minutes. Smaller goals are achievable. Achievable goals are reached.

- Walk. It's the best advice any busy, working person can get. For the majority of my clients, walking becomes the mainstay of their exercise program. Many of my commuter clients find that they can walk to or from the train on their daily commute. You can park farther from your destination (and save time searching endlessly for that close space!) and benefit from the longer walk. If you take a bus or subway, you can get off a stop or two early and enjoy the fresh air and the walk.

- Climb stairs. Before there was a StairMaster, there were actual stairs! You just walked up them! You can still do this in your office. Many people sit almost all day long. So unless you're in a building that discourages use of the stairway, make a point of doing two or four flights of stairs a couple of times a day. You'll be surprised at how quickly and effectively it can get your heart rate up, relieve stress, and of course, burn calories.

- Bring it indoors. If the roads are too icy to run and you've just about had it with all the layers of clothing, let winter provide the opportunity to try new indoor exercise options: power yoga, Pilates, spin classes, home exercise tapes, dance classes. The bottom line: keep moving. Any exercise is better than nothing, and you can't eat while you're exercising!

- Change your exercise routine. A new routine works an entirely new set of muscles. You'll be sore the first few days, I promise. Changing your exercise routine allows your overworked muscles to rest, and it often gets you out of a workout rut.

- If your budget allows, consider getting a personal trainer. Busy people often find that having a trainer scheduled into their week ensures that exercise will be part of their regular routine. A trainer can also advise you in your choice of exercises and can help you exercise effectively so you get the best results with the least chance of injury or strain. And bear in mind that you don't have to use a trainer for a long period of time; if you prefer, you can simply consult with someone a few times to get you started.

- If you're ready to advance from the Twenty-Minute Rule, spinning is a good exercise for busy people. Many of my Wall Street clients enjoy it. It's ordinarily a forty-five-minute class that requires a huge burst of energy. It boosts your heart rate and gives you an intense exercise session in a relatively short time.

- Wii your way to weight loss. Nintendo Wii is an interactive game with options that will actually get you off your duff and include tennis, boxing, etc. I have one client who claimed she hated to exercise, but she recently reported that she and her husband now play Wii every night for an hour. This is an especially good option for dads who want an activity they can enjoy with their kids when they get home from work.

- Try iTrain. ITrain programs are audio MP3 files that combine Hollywood personal trainer workouts and music entertainment. Learn more at *www.itrain.com.*

I hope you've been inspired to look for more information on exercise if you don't already exercise regularly. And if exercise is already a part of your regular routine, I know that the Wall Street Diet, combined with your physical activity, is going to make an appreciable difference in your efforts to lose weight.

The Wall Street
Closing Statement

L et's take a look at a few of the issues that can pop up when you're
working on your weight. Of course, it's not always smooth sailing and
many of my clients need advice, as time goes on, on how to deal with
plateaus and maintenance issues. And everybody needs a morale boost
now and again, so that's what this chapter is about.

Plateaus

*"Heather refers to weight as decades. At 170, I was 'a 70s gal' des-
perate to get to the 60s. But nothing was happening. Heather told me
that in her experience this was partly because I'd dieted often in the
past. Seems I'm a slow loser. What helped me to stick with it was that
I was looking and feeling better. I just had to cross my fingers and
believe and keep doing the diet. Sure enough, twelve more days and
suddenly three pounds were gone. Heather was right; I'm glad I was
patient."*

—PAULA B., HEADMISTRESS, MANHATTAN PRIVATE SCHOOL

It's almost inevitable. You've done a great job on your diet. You've really turned the corner and your clothes are looser and you're feeling great. You've lost eight pounds. So why can't you make it ten? Even after two weeks of careful dieting? Plateaus are an annoying fact of diet life. The simple truth is that weight loss is always erratic. Always. Diets that promise otherwise just aren't telling the truth. You may quickly lose five or ten pounds and then get stuck for a week with absolutely no results. I've found this to be particularly true of people who are stressed. I'm not sure if this is due to elevated levels of cortisol—the stress hormone—or other hormone or thyroid issues. It may explain why people seem to lose weight on vacation, or at least don't gain, even when they're eating more than usual. I do know that I've seen some very erratic patterns in weight loss among my clients over the years. You need to respect your own metabolism and how long it takes for you to lose weight and stabilize. Remember that you're built to respond to different levels of calorie intake: reduced calorie intake is going to change your metabolism and the rate at which you burn calories and lose weight. Men, in particular, seem to get stuck around two hundred pounds. Somehow that number seems to be a hurdle. It's not unusual for a client to come to me and say, "It's not working. I haven't lost a pound in over a week." I tell my clients, "It is working. Don't your clothes feel looser than a week ago? Don't you *feel* like you're losing weight? Just promise me that you'll give it one more week." It always works. Sometimes people will go ten days or two weeks without losing an ounce and then I'll get a little ping on my BlackBerry: "Heather, I'm down three pounds this morning!"

The scale can sometimes be an enemy. The hardest thing for a dieter to do, especially after a few weeks of success, is to hold fast through a plateau. Here are some strategies to help you break through:

- **RECORD.** This is the single most useful strategy for those who get stuck. It's human nature to relax a bit after you've had some success with weight loss. But if you want to continue to lose, you have to tighten it up. Record what you're eating and you may be surprised. Most people know what to eat in front of others. They'd never order the fettuccine Alfredo or an ice cream sundae. But they succumb to nibbles throughout the day and don't count them. Sometimes clients complain of being stalled, but their food journals tell the story: a cookie from the receptionist's desk, a few wings after work. It all counts, but you can't count it if you pretend it's not happening!

- Are you hungry at bedtime? Not ravenous but just a bit hungry. Are you hungry in the morning? If you want to continue to lose weight, you may have to feel hungry at one of these two times.

- Decrease your total weekly Juicy Carb intake by one or two.

- If you've been following the ¾ Rule—eating three-quarters of the food on your plate—shift to half for a few days.

- Add a Veggie Night. If you haven't been doing any, add one. If you've been doing one, add another. (See pages 88–89.)

- Do one or two Protein Days in one week. (See pages 87–88.)

- Shift your frozen dinner selections to those under 300 calories. Most people don't notice this change in terms of their satisfaction after eating, but their scale will.

- Try an omelet dinner. A four-egg-white omelet with some vegetables is satisfying and very low in calories.

- Drink more water. Add one 20-ounce bottle of water daily.

- Take baby steps: Do you sweeten your coffee or tea? If so, try to skip the sweetener for a week (or at least use less). If you are drinking diet soda, try to cut it out or at least reduce the amount you drink. These changes have actually helped clients break past a plateau.

- Are you having a Fun Snack every day? If so, try to skip it for three days a week. If it's too hard for you to skip the snack and your snack is a bar, choose a lower-calorie bar. For example, switch from the 190-calorie Lärabar to a 110-calorie Pria bar. Alternatively, try changing from a bar to a piece of fruit. Just those few calories could help boost you off your plateau in a few days.

- Add ten to twenty minutes onto your exercise routine if you have one. If you don't have one, try to boost your physical activity in whatever way you can. This can make a big difference in your weight loss.

- Pay attention to volume. If you're eating cereal or yogurt, make sure the amounts are appropriate.

BEWARE THE AFTERSHOCK *Just as the weight can come off erratically, so it can creep back up with its own inexplicable timing. Maybe you've experienced this. You've lost weight; you're feeling great. So you have a nibble here, a treat there. It's all OK; you're still at your goal weight. A week goes by and you get on the scale, and seemingly overnight—kaboom!—you're three pounds up! What the heck? I call this the Aftershock. Your body is not a simple machine. And you can't fool it. Your body can take a while to catch up to your bad habits, but it will eventually. The Aftershock is how most people gain weight. They're thin for a while and they get cocky. They begin to eat junk, forget about exercising, and think it's all fine, they're still thin. And then one day: bam—fifteen pounds!! So beware the Aftershock!*

Maintenance

It's all over when the fat lady is no longer fat! But getting there is one thing; staying there is another. Successful dieters recognize that they're in it for the long haul. Remember that it's not a sprint; it's a marathon. As I mentioned in the Introduction to this book, I'm proud of all my clients, but the ones who really win my heart are those who bounce up and down a bit but overall keep their weight off. To me, that's a real success. So be patient with yourself and you will get where you want to be. And once you do . . .

Maintenance is the term that most diets use for the phase when the dieter has reached a goal and wants to stay there, or move to another level. Before we explore the Wall Street Maintenance Guidelines, I'd like you to consider a couple of things about your goal weight. For one thing, many people have a sort of fantasy weight that floats in their head. The fantasy is that when they reach that number, they'll have reached nirvana. Don't let yourself get too tied to "the number." Of course your weight is important, and it's good to measure progress, but your personal "ideal" weight isn't carved in stone. Some clients have proposed a goal weight that they later realized was unrealistic. They found they were happy and looked great at a slightly higher number. Remember, too, that your weight fluctuates. Most people's weight floats within a few pounds day to day and that's normal and nothing to focus on. As long as you're in the vicinity of where you'd like to be, you're doing great.

Reached your goal weight? Fantastic! But in my book you haven't really reached your goal until you've stayed at or around that weight for a month. A month? What's that about? you may ask. Well, I've seen too many clients start to party the day they reach their goal weight. It's akin to the diets that clients tell me about where you can take a "day off." This almost never works because people just have a "Might-as-Well" day that slips into another "Might-as-Well" day, and before you know it, it's game over! The Wall Street Diet is a lifestyle diet, and so it's not about reaching a goal and going wild! Once you've reached your goal, you should go into a goal holding pattern. Stick with what you've been doing and prove to yourself that you've actually accomplished quite a lot.

And now to the maintenance details . . . Frankly, many of my clients are somewhat loose about maintenance. They are very careful about what they eat, and if they see they're up a pound or two or if their clothes get a bit tight, they cut back. Others want very strict rules and guidelines on what they should eat once they reach their desired weight. My guidelines on how to carry on once you've reached your goal are fairly simple. They include five points:

1. When you've stayed at your weight loss goal for a month, you can increase your total Juicy Carb intake. So:

    • If you're having four Juicy Carbs a week, you can bump it up to seven, so you'll be having seven a week or one each day.

- If you're already having one Juicy Carb a day, you can now have two a day.

2. You can add two Pleasures a week if you like. Each Pleasure counts as a Juicy Carb. I'll explain below about the Pleasure. Some people don't have any for a week or two and then two in one week. It's your choice.

3. Think about changing your snacks when you reach Maintenance. Check the list of Fun Snacks (pages 311–12) for some new ideas.

4. Try a new soup or sandwich. Many people stick to their salads or protein/veggies until they reach their goal, so adding in a soup option, a turkey sandwich on whole wheat or rye, or a new frozen dinner can feel luxurious.

5. Choose a different breakfast. See pages 209–210 for Maintenance Breakfast suggestions.

THE SCARY TRUTH ABOUT SMOKED SALMON *Many clients ask if they can choose smoked salmon as a protein option for breakfast. As it has only about 100 calories for three ounces, it seems, at first blush, like a reasonable choice. But the salmon calories are only half the story here. Most smoked salmon has roughly 1700 mg of sodium per 3 ounces (calories and sodium vary depending on the type of salmon and how it's smoked). So an excess of sodium is almost guaranteed. But it gets worse: most people eat far more than 3 ounces of salmon at a sitting. I've also seen bagel stores in Manhattan add as much as 9 ounces of salmon to a single order (that would be 297 calories and a whopping 5100 mg of sodium). When you add a bagel at 350 calories, you're up 647 calories! So here's my Wall Street Diet version of a smoked salmon breakfast: 1 slice of salmon (BlackBerry size) on top of 2 Fiber Rich crackers with 2 T of 1% Friendship whipped cottage cheese, cucumber, tomato, and onion. This is only appropriate for a Maintenance Breakfast.*

It's All About the Pleasures

The Pleasures are the enjoyable foods that you can reintroduce into your diet because your weight is now stable. Pick your Pleasure! You can have two Pleasures a week. A pleasure is an indulgence that counts as one Juicy Carb. It can be anything—a dessert, an extra glass of wine—whatever food treat would please you. The only important thing you need to remember about your Pleasure is that it must be a normal serving: a bowl of ice cream is fine; a pint of ice cream is not. A roll from the bread basket is fine; half of a baguette is not. Some restaurant servings or commercial foods (I'm looking at you, Cheescake Factory!) are not normal portions, and I'm sure you'll be able to recognize those. Usually a Pleasure is best enjoyed with other people, and there should be no guilt associated with it. It's all about mindful indulgence. You deserve it; you earned it; enjoy it! Some Pleasures that clients enjoy include a bagel in the morning (if you're a Controlled Eater), a burger with fries at lunch, perhaps a child-sized popcorn at the movies, or an appetizer-sized portion of a pasta dish you've been longing for.

A few guidelines on the Pleasures include:

- If you're a Clean Plate Club Eater, a Pleasure may be a food trigger for you, so I suggest you save your Pleasures for evening—dessert after dinner.

- If you're a Controlled Eater, you can enjoy your Pleasure at almost any time of day, so long as it doesn't trigger overeating. If a beer at lunch sets you off, then it's best to have it in the evening.

- Portion sizes really count with Pleasures. Don't fool yourself. A giant honking bag of popcorn is not a Pleasure; it's a Dirty Deed!

- When the Pleasure is finished, it's over! You're right back on track with your regular Wall Street choices. Actually, most clients tell me that they've grown so accustomed to their routine foods that it's not a big deal to stay with them.

- Pleasures are all about . . . well, pleasure! Enjoy them! Don't dare feel guilty about them. Food is one of the joys of living and you're meant to savor it.

AVOID THE RED ZONE *I tell my clients to watch out for the Red Zone. Once you reach your goal weight, or a weight you're happy with, if you go five pounds above that number, you're in the Red Zone and you need to pull yourself back. Sometimes this happens when you stop weighing your-self. Sometimes it's just two bad days in a row or a bad weekend. The best thing to do if you hit the Red Zone is a Protein Day. That will get you back on track. Remember, anyone can slip into the Red Zone; no one should stay there!*

Maintenance Breakfasts

In general, your meals, except for your added Pleasures, stay the same on Maintenance. The only difference is at breakfast when there is a host of new options you can choose from.

Some of these breakfasts count as a Juicy Carb (JC); some don't.

The additional Maintenance Breakfast Options are (all are listed on the Shopping List, pages 305–6):

- **WAFFLES:** 2 Kashi Go Lean or Van's organic original waffles (plain or blueberry) with ½ cup berries, ½ cup whipped cottage cheese, and 1 teaspoon sugar-free syrup. This makes a nice weekend breakfast. (JC)

- Amy's frozen breakfast choices: Amy's Breakfast Burrito; Amy's Tofu Scramble Pocket; 2 Amy's Breakfast Patties plus 1 Fiber Rich cracker and 1 fruit; Amy's Toaster Pop plus 1 Laughing Cow Light cheese. (The toaster pop is like a pop tart, but it is organic and obviously much healthier. You can choose the calorie count you prefer on these. Just check the packages: the burrito is almost 300 calories and the tofu scramble pocket is 180 calories; you can check out all the products at *www.amys.com*.) (JC)

- Veggie links/sausage: 2 MorningStar Veggie Links plus 2 Fiber Rich, plus 1 fruit. Or 2 Al Fresco apple-maple chicken sausages. (There are other sausage brand options on the Shopping List, page 307, including Casual Gourmet and Bilinski's, and yes, they will all be plus 2 Fiber Rich and a fruit.)

- Boca Meatless Breakfast Wrap plus one optional fruit. (JC)

- Switch out any Fiber Rich in a breakfast above with Thomas' Light Multi-Grain English Muffin. (JC)

- Vitamuffin with 1 Laughing Cow Light cheese wedge (make sure this is the muffin top or the 2-ounce muffin that is 100 calories). (JC)

- Breakfast burrito: Low-carb wrap—either La Tortilla, Mission Carb Balance Wrap, Trader Joe's Low-Carb Wrap, or Damascus Bakeries Whole Wheat Roll Up (counts as a fiber at breakfast) plus egg whites or Egg Beaters with veggies, Laughing Cow Light cheese, 1 tablespoon salsa, and ¼ cup avocado chunks.

- Thomas' Light Multi-Grain English Muffin toasted with ½ cup Friendship whipped cottage cheese and 1 tablespoon Smucker's sugar-free preserves. (JC)

Vacation

A vacation is a vacation from everything except eating well. I urge my Wall Street clients to get out there and really savor their vacations. It isn't a time to count cheese wedges and skip a glass of wine, even at lunch! But there's no reason to go whole hog, and in fact almost every client has told me that they miss their regular foods when they're away. They really have no trouble eating well, and they normally find when they get home that they've stayed the same weight or even lost weight.

Here are the Wall Street Vacation Guidelines:

- **NO MATTER WHAT YOU'VE BEEN DOING BEFORE YOU LEAVE:** You can have two Juicy Carbs a day. Save them for lunch/dinner or both at dinner. You can have one Pleasure a day at dinner, and it counts as the Juicy Carb. All protein, fruit, veggies, and fat are *free* on vacation; do not worry about portion control or how the food is prepared. Alcohol will not count as your Juicy Carb.

- **BEFORE YOUR TRIP:** If you are going to be away for a long time, you can bring some food with you—Fiber Rich crackers, Justin's Nut Butter, and uncoated bars (Luna Toasted Nuts 'n Cranberry). Alternatively you can simply go empty-handed and relax a bit. Vacation is a nice break from life and your current food options; you'll look forward to enjoying your regular cereal, Fun Snacks, and crackers when you get home. If you're going away for a short time—a week or less—I don't think you should worry about bringing food. Just relax and enjoy your time off. If you eat reasonably well and exercise, you will be able to keep any extra pounds at bay.

- **BREAKFAST:** Whether you have a continental or full breakfast included in your hotel or are going out of your hotel to eat, there are a few staples that can be found anywhere. Eggs and omelets (egg whites are even better) are always a great choice and will keep you full for a long time. Whole grain cereal with either skim milk or yogurt is also good. Add a piece of fruit with these choices. An easy breakfast rule for travelers that makes their diet easier: always skip the Dry Carb at breakfast. You're probably not sure of what the rest of your day will bring, but if you can get off to a good Dry-Carb-Free morning, you're already ahead of the competition.

- **LUNCH:** When you're traveling, the most common lunchtime options are salads, soups, and sandwiches. Do not automatically choose an unappetizing salad (say, at a museum café) just because you think it is healthier. In that instance, go for the delicious-looking sandwich. If the sandwich is on a huge baguette that's too big to fit in your mouth, take off the top piece of bread. If you are at a sit-down lunch, order an entrée salad, but forgo the bread and alcohol because it would be better to save your carb for dinner. A broth-based soup and a small salad is another great option.

- **DINNER:** On vacation you want to indulge a little, but you want to be selective. You are going to choose what you want the *most*. Maybe the bread in France is what you crave, or maybe you want to split a pasta appetizer in Italy, or a dessert anywhere, or have a glass or two of wine. Just remember, indulging is OK, but try to share if you can and order healthily for the other parts of the meal. If you want to split a dessert, get a mixed green salad to start, a lean protein entrée with vegetables, and then get the dessert. If you are craving steak frites, then order it but skip bread and dessert.

Personal Power

I've noticed over the years as I've worked with people who struggle to lose weight that an often-overlooked factor in a dieter's success is their personal grooming. It may sound frivolous, but I've invariably found it to be true: when you spend some time on yourself—on making yourself look better—you feel better about yourself and you feel empowered. This sense of power helps you stick to your food goals and reach success. I thought it would be useful and reassuring to you to give you some suggestions on little ways you can reinforce the positive way you feel when you start to lose weight.

- **DRESS FOR SUCCESS.** Sometimes people who have been overweight hide in their clothes. When you begin to get trimmer, showing off your body only makes you feel better about what you've achieved. Make time to buy a new suit for work or some more fitted and fashionable weekend clothes. You'd be surprised how loose-fitting clothes can be a deterrent to weight loss. More fitted clothes=less room to eat!

- **DISCOVER UNDERCOVER CONFIDENCE.** Men: get rid of those stretched-out old shorts or boxers. You'll feel more complete with a fresh set. Women: a small investment in sexy lingerie can be highly motivating. There's nothing like a thong to help keep your mind off pastry. You'll wear your clothes better and you'll feel better.

- **A POLISHED HANDSHAKE SEALS THE DEAL.** Your hands work hard in business and people notice them. They're visible all the time—at meetings, while entertaining. A beautiful manicure makes you seem like someone who has everything under control. You can mani-*cure* your hunger! And men shouldn't be afraid of a manicure. A few of my male clients get a manicure just so they can enjoy the shoulder massage at the end. Hands on the levers of power should look good.

- **TRIM HAIR, TRIM BODY.** Did you ever notice that you eat better the day that your hair's freshly styled? Men should grab time regularly for a trim and a shave at the barbershop. Ladies can get a blow-out between regular hair stylings. It's relaxing and it boosts confidence to know you look great, and it makes it so much easier to pass on dessert.

- **DITCH THE "QUITTERS."** Men: you probably have a drawer half-full of quitters. Quitters are those falling down socks that, like a pebble in your shoe, distract and annoy you. Invest in a set of fresh, new, hardworking socks. You'll feel pulled together and on top of the world.

- **THE IMELDA MARCOS DIET TIP.** New shoes! Ladies, forget that high heels make your legs look slim and that you love the way they look. Keep in mind that the extra height they give you is empowering and even, sometimes (when you need it to be), intimidating. So indulge in a couple of pairs of sexy shoes. You can walk in your walking shoes; use your stilettos as "meeting shoes."

- **TAKE A SHINE TO YOUR FEET.** Men: A shoe shine polishes your whole look and gives you a new lease on life. It also gives you a pause in your busy day and the opportunity to sit on a throne. What's not to like?

- **SWEAT IT OUT.** There is nothing like a good sweat to renew and refresh you. It's a time-honored healthy practice. Find an opportunity to indulge in a steam bath at your local gym or hotel. Or try a Bikram Yoga (or Hot Yoga) class. You'll feel like a new you.

"Only four weeks or so after I began seeing Heather Bauer my friends began asking, 'What happened to YOU?' I wasn't sure what they meant, but suddenly they were ALL asking for Heather's card—even my cardiologist! She is famous now in my circle as 'the answer' to the yo-yo diet syndrome. I am so very grateful to have found her, and so are my friends. I never dreamed that at my age, post-menopause, I could be as thin as I am now. She is definitely the answer, as my doctor confirms, to the middle-aged woman's longing for her figure of the past. Well, with Heather, it is all possible. She also knows all the restaurants in town and helps her clients plan meals out. She is the most remarkable, even extraordinary, nutritionist I have ever consulted—and so say all of my [skinny yet healthy] friends."

—DR. KRISTIN O. LAUER, PROFESSOR, FORDHAM UNIVERSITY

PART IV

The Wall Street Cheat Sheets

Here is a wealth of information on how to eat on the road, whether you're grabbing lunch or breakfast at your corner deli, eating with the kids at a fast-food place, choosing an appetizer at a high-end hotel bar, grabbing a drink at a sports bar, or settling in for a double feature at the movies. We've also included some suggestions on how to work the salad bar, as well as some original salad bar "recipes" that will lift your greens out of the doldrums. Finally, there's the Wall Street Shopping List. It's a complete list, with websites where appropriate, of all the foods suggested on the Wall Street Diet.

Beverages

Alcoholic Drink Picks and Skips

PICK	CALORIES
Glass of red or white wine (4 oz)	80–85
Light beer (12 oz)	99
White wine spritzer	45
Vodka and soda (or diet tonic)	100
Scotch on the rocks	100

SKIP	CALORIES
Margarita	300
Egg nog	305
Piña colada	465

Calories in Common Drinks

	SIZE (OZ.)	CALORIES
BEER		
Low-Carb Beer	12	96
Light Beer	12	99
Beer (regular)	12	146
Stout (Guinness)	16 (1 pint)	170
WINE		
White Wine	4	80
Red Wine	4	85
Dessert Wine	4	181
White Wine Spritzer (½ wine/½ seltzer)	5	45
Sake	4	160
Champagne	4	85–90
SPIRITS		
Vodka (80 proof)	1.5	100
Scotch	1.5	100
Gin (80 proof)	1.5	100
Rum (80 proof)	1.5	100
Tequila (80 proof)	1.5	100
Whiskey (80 proof)	1.5	100
MIXERS		
Club Soda	6	0
Diet Soda (or Diet Tonic)	8	0
Soda (Coke)	8	105
Red Bull	8	113
Orange Juice	8	120
Pineapple Juice	8	150
Tonic	6	178
Cranberry Juice	6	190
POPULAR MIXED DRINKS		
Rum and Diet Coke	8	100–110
Vodka and Soda (or Diet Tonic)	8	100–110

	SIZE (OZ.)	CALORIES

POPULAR MIXED DRINKS (CONTINUED)

	SIZE (OZ.)	CALORIES
Whiskey Sour	3	122
Bloody Mary	5	125–140
Mojito	5	143
Martini (no olives)	3	190
Rum and Coke	8	205–240
Gin and Tonic	5	210
Manhattan	3.5	210
Martini (with olives)	3	220
Daiquiri	4	222
Vodka Cranberry	8	250–290
Margarita	8	300
Egg Nog	5	305
Piña Colada	8	465

Coffee Bar Picks and Skips

For all coffee/tea choices the best option is hot or cold tea or coffee for 0–5 calories (no additions). If the calories in the drink exceed 60, you must lower the calories in your breakfast to compensate (or add fruit and count it as a breakfast if they're over 150). For an occasional afternoon Fun Snack you can pick a drink under 200 calories. *Note*: All recommended picks are Tall sizes (or ounces are specified). If you choose a larger size, pay attention to the additional calories.

Starbucks

HOT DRINKS

PICK (ALL TALL)	CALORIES
Brewed Tazo Teas	0
Brewed coffee/Caffe Americano (before milk)	5–10
Espresso (solo)	5
Nonfat cappuccino (best to order extra dry)	60
Nonfat Caffè Misto	60

Heather's hot beverage recipe: Venti Tea with 2 Chai tea bags, some skim, and a Splenda (estimated 30 calories)

SKIP (BOTH VENTI)	CALORIES
Caffè Mocha (whole milk, with whipped cream)	450
Caramel Macchiato (whole milk)	340

COLD DRINKS

PICK (ALL TALL)	CALORIES
Iced coffee (freshly brewed over ice, no milk)	5
Nonfat Iced Sugar-Free Vanilla Latte	60
Frappuccino Light Blended Coffee (various flavors)	110–140

Heather's cold beverage recipe: Venti size, ½ iced green tea, ½ lemonade (request no syrup), and add your own Splenda (estimated 60 calories)

SKIP (BOTH VENTI)	CALORIES
Java Chip Frappuccino Blended Crème (with whipped cream)	600
Double Chocolate Chip Blended Crème (whole milk, with whipped cream)	670

The Coffee Beanery

HOT DRINKS

PICK	CALORIES
Tea	0
Beanery Blend Coffee (before milk or sugar)	2
Sugar-Free Caffi Mocha Tall with Skim Milk (12 oz)	80
Cappuccino (Tall)	130

SKIP	CALORIES
Hot Cocoa (Tall)	340
Caramelatte Tall (12 oz)	390
Caramelatte Grande (16 oz)	490

COLD DRINKS

PICK	CALORIES
Iced coffee with added skim (Tall)	30
Iced Café Latte (Tall)	130
Iced Cappuccino (Tall)	130
Tea-Wave Smoothie (8 oz, various flavors)	136–169

SKIP	CALORIES
Caramel Frappalatte (20 oz)	420
White Mocha Frappalatte (20 oz)	460

Dunkin' Donuts

HOT DRINKS

PICK	CALORIES
Tea	0
Coffee (black, 10 oz)	15
Any flavored coffee (hazelnut, French vanilla, etc., before milk)	20
Coffee (with skim milk, 10 oz)	25
Vanilla Latte Lite (10 oz)	80

SKIP	CALORIES
Gingerbread Latte (10 oz)	400
White Hot Chocolate (14 oz)	340
Caramel Crème Hot Latte (10 oz)	260

COLD DRINKS

PICK	CALORIES
Iced coffee with skim milk (16 oz)	25
Iced Latte with skim milk (16 oz)	70
Turbo Ice (16 oz)	120

SKIP	CALORIES
Mango Passion Fruits Smoothie (24 oz)	550
Tropical Fruit Smoothie Small (16 oz)	360
Strawberry Fruit Coolatta (16 oz)	290

Peet's Coffee & Tea

HOT DRINKS

PICK	CALORIES
Small tea, no milk	0
Small coffee, no milk	5
Small cappuccino with fat-free milk (12 oz)	68
Small latte with fat-free milk (12 oz)	101
Small latte macchiato with fat-free milk (12 oz)	101

SKIP	CALORIES
Small white chocolate mocha with whipped cream (12 oz)	398
Large latte with whole milk (20 oz)	263

COLD DRINKS

PICK	CALORIES
Iced tea	0
Iced coffee	5
Iced latte with fat-free milk (12 oz)	101

SKIP	CALORIES
Medium Scharffen Berger Chocolate Mocha Freddo with whipped cream (16 oz)	420
Large Caffe Freddo without whipped cream (20 oz)	331

IN GENERAL, AVOID

- All venti-sized beverages (24 oz for cold drinks, 20 oz for hot)

- Beverages made with whole milk

Buffet, Bar, and Deli Meal Picks and Skips

I t's a real challenge to select wisely when you are confronted with a relatively limitless array of food. But you can make good choices if you know the best options. Here are some guidelines for how to make the best picks in a host of all-you-can-eat situations, as well as some guidelines for deli lunches.*

---

* Recipes and serving sizes vary, so calorie amounts are provided in ranges and as estimates for many of the items within this section.

Breakfast Buffets

PICK	CALORIES
Fruit salad (approx 1 cup)	75–150
Hard-boiled egg	75
Egg-white omelet (with Pam, 1–3 veggies) (Add additional 50–100 calories for omelet made with regular oil.)	100–175
Cereal (Kellogg's for example) in mini box with ½ cup skim milk	120–150
Oatmeal (1 c)	100–150
Bacon (2 strips, pan-fried)	70–82
Canadian bacon (about 2 slices)	70–90
Yogurt (1 cup, ideally light or nonfat)	60–150
2 poached eggs	150
Scrambled eggs (about 2 eggs)	150–200
Wheat toast with jam	100–150

SKIP	CALORIES
Biscuit (large, without butter)	300
Muffins (large, 4–5 oz)	300–500
Scones	450–500
Large bagel with regular cream cheese	550
Pancakes (4) with syrup (¼ c)	870
Belgian waffle with fruit and whipped cream	900

Lunch and Deli Meals

PICK	CALORIES
¼ container low-fat tuna salad	140
¼ container low-fat chicken salad	200
¼ lb turkey breast and a small fruit salad	180–220
Veggie sandwich on whole wheat (2 cups veggies)	170–200
Turkey on whole wheat bread with lettuce and tomato (4 oz turkey)	240–280
Chicken breast on whole wheat bread with lettuce and tomato (4 oz chicken)	240–300
Ham on whole wheat bread with lettuce and tomato (4 oz ham)	260–340

NOTE:

- Calorie estimates do not include condiments; always choose regular mustard.

- Low-fat tuna and chicken salad are made with low-fat mayo.

	CALORIES
Chicken noodle soup (bowl)	80
Minestrone soup (bowl)	80
Tomato vegetable (bowl)	90

NOTE:

- Calorie estimates for soup vary depending on size. Minestrone and chicken noodle typically count as a Juicy Carb for the day. If soup has beans or lentils in it and that is the protein for the meal, no Juicy Carb is used. Those who are salt-sensitive should skip soup option.

SKIP	CALORIES
Bologna on a plain wrap (4 oz bologna)	610–670
Salami on a plain wrap (4 oz salami)	570–650
Cheese on a plain wrap (4 oz cheese)	670–720+
Tuna salad (with regular mayo) on a plain wrap	570–670

NOTE:

- Plain wrap estimated at 310 calories.

- Calorie estimates do not include condiments, vegetables, or cheese.

Broccoli cheddar soup (1 c)	350–400
Split pea with ham (1 c)	350
Shrimp bisque (1 c)	300

Hors D'Oeuvres and Cocktail Party Food

PICK	CALORIES
Sushi (1 piece California roll)	30–40
(1 piece Cucumber roll)	20–25
Shrimp cocktail (2 boiled shrimp + 2 tsp cocktail sauce)	50
Veggies with salsa (10 veggie slices + 2 T salsa)	50
Osetra caviar (1 oz)	75
Grilled mini lamb chops (1)	80
Veggie spring roll (steamed, 2 pieces)	50–140
Veggie crudite (10 veggie slices + 1 T full-fat dip)	100–125
Chicken satay (2 skewers)	100
Bruschetta with tomato and basil (1 piece)	110
Shrimp dumplings (steamed, 3 dumplings)	130
Mushroom crostini* (2–3 pieces)	140
Mushroom and gruyere tartlets (2 pieces)	140
Deviled eggs (2 halves)	120–150
Pot stickers with soy ginger sauce (2 pieces, 2T sauce)	150

SKIP	CALORIES
Egg roll (fried, pork, 1 egg roll, medium-sized)	240
Stuffed clams (3 small)	270
Mini pizza (5 small)	260–300
Pigs in blankets (cocktail franks, 4 pieces)	270
Bacon-wrapped figs (4 pieces)	280
Swedish meatballs (2 pieces/3 oz)	300
Mini spring rolls (fried, 2 pieces + 1 T sauce)	320

* Crostini includes mushrooms, dip, and French bread slices.

Sports Bars and Bar and Grills

WALL STREET TIPS FOR MEALS AT ANY BAR AND GRILL–TYPE RESTAURANT

- Consider soup and salad or burger/sandwich with no bread and a house salad.

- Opt for broth-based soups (such as vegetable or chicken noodle) instead of cream-based soups.

- Ask for a side salad or side veggie instead of French fries or onion rings.

- Most bar and grill restaurants offer a basic garden salad and are willing to add grilled chicken if requested.

- Ask about salad dressing options and choose light or fat-free options. If none are available, select a vinaigrette.

- Modify sandwich options to make healthier by omitting cheese and bacon and by selecting mustard instead of mayo.

- Avoid dishes that have the words "crunchy" or "crispy" in the name. This usually means fried. Look for "baked," "grilled," "blackened," or "roasted" instead.

PICK	CALORIES
Chicken noodle soup (bowl)	100–200
Chili (cup)	180
Vegetable soup (bowl)	220
House/garden salad with low-fat/fat-free dressing	150–300
Hamburger on bun (no cheese, no sides)	350–600
Hamburger patty without bun (no cheese, no sides)	200–450
Grilled chicken sandwich (no sides, no cheese) with mustard	300–450
Grilled chicken breast without bun (no sides, no cheese)	150–300

SKIP	CALORIES
Cheese fries with creamy/cheesy dressing	2070
Chicken quesadilla	1830
Classic nachos with pico de gallo and sour cream	1450
Buffalo wings with blue cheese dressing (10 wings)	1340
Mozzarella sticks with marinara sauce (9 sticks)	1210

Bar Snacks

This is the horror show for dieters. Take a deep breath and just one glance down at the list of Skips I've listed here. Yes, it's a long list. It's meant to frighten you. You can see that a couple of hours of munching bar snacks could set you way back on your weight loss goal. This is why I often suggest that clients simply make a bar visit their dinner: skip the snacks and have a burger (no fries!) and a salad and be done with it. Now you won't be able to say you didn't know.

PICK	CALORIES
Vegetable crudite, no dip (calories vary depending on amount)	25–75

SKIP	CALORIES
5 pretzels	60
1 handful M&M's	129
4 crackers with 1 oz cheese	140
1 handful honey-roasted peanuts (1 oz)	160
5 pieces of a California roll	180
12 candy-coated almonds	230
4–5 handfuls Wasabi peas (3 oz)	260
2 handfuls Chex Mix (2 oz)	246
Tortilla chips (12–15 chips)	140
1 cup guacamole	367
Nachos (small order, cheese only)	350–400
4 mozzarella sticks	431
3 martinis	480
Wings (5 wings with 3 T blue cheese dressing)	500–600
8 potato chips with dip	600
6 nachos (with beans, cheese, and ground beef)	569
with sour cream and guacamole it is 150 calories more	719
Mixed nuts (1 c, 5–6 handfuls)	875

Best Picks from Popular New York Sports Bars

Every town has its popular watering holes. I wanted to give you a sample of the offerings at a couple of New York spots to give you a general idea of the calorie range in common food choices.

P.J. Clarke's

PICK	CALORIES
French onion soup (ask for no cheese or croutons)	80–120
Mixed greens	100–150
Irish beef barley soup	150–200
Shrimp cocktail	200–300
PEI steamed mussels for two (share with another person)	200–300
Classic Caesar (ask for dressing on the side, use 2 T)	250–350
Andy Boy Broccoli Rabe	100–150
Sauteed button mushrooms	100–150

Blondies Sports Bar and Restaurant

PICK	CALORIES
Chicken vegetable soup (skip the garlic parmesan bread)	100–150
Italian Wedding Soup (skip the garlic parmesan bread)	100–150
Fresh-cut fruit (served with cottage cheese or low-fat yogurt, ½ cup of either)	150–250
Broccoli, green peppers, zucchini, carrots, and celery with spinach dip (order a small platter, use 2 tsp dip)	100–200
Sauteed vegetables	100–150
Marinated grilled shrimp (5) (use about 2T of cocktail sauce)	200–250
Blondies Chopped Salad with or without grilled chicken (ask for no cheddar or bacon, and use 2 T fat-free balsamic roasted garlic or sun-dried tomato-basil dressing)	300–400

Upscale Hotel Bar Food Picks and Skips

PICK	CALORIES
Shrimp cocktail (6 boiled shrimp + 2 T cocktail sauce)	150
Tuna sushi/sashimi/tartar options	50–200
Caesar salads (with chicken or lobster, no dressing)	150–350

SKIP	CALORIES
Crab cakes (1)	290
Crispy popcorn shrimp (1 serving)	300–500
9-oz burger (90% lean ground beef broiled is 180 cals/3 oz)	540+
Turkey club (full sandwich with bacon and mayo)	1000
BBQ baby back ribs (per serving at Chilis)	800–1200

Best Picks from Popular Hotel Bars in Manhattan

Church Lounge at the Tribeca Grand Hotel

Kitchen is willing to accommodate dietary restrictions or preferences, including low-fat/allergies.

PICK	CALORIES
Shrimp ceviche (green olives, tomato, capers, and oregano)	150–350
Tuna tartare	250–450
Miso Chilean Sea Bass Skewers	200–400

Rise at the Ritz-Carlton Hotel "Light Fare Menu"

PICK	CALORIES
Seared Satés (platter of 5, split with a friend, order the chicken)	100–200
Jumbo shrimp cocktail horseradish tomato sauce	200–300

King Cole Bar & Lounge at the St. Regis Hotel

PICK	CALORIES
Vidalia Onion Soup	80–120
East Coast Oysters	50–150
Chicken Saté	100–150
Colossal Shrimp Cocktail	200–300

Gilt at the New York Palace Hotel

PICK	CALORIES
Yellow Fin Tuna Tartare	250–450
Tomato sauce and Black Olive Tapenade	100–300
Chilled oysters on the half shell (18)	50–150

Pen-Top Bar & Terrace at the Peninsula Hotel

PICK	CALORIES
Marinated shrimp cocktail	200–300
Sushi and sashimi platter	200–400

Sporting Events and Concession Stands

PICK	CALORIES
Fruit cup (6 oz)	70
Veggie cup (8 oz)	70
Garden burger/Boca burgers (without bun)	90–150
Vegan/turkey burger (cooked, 4 oz)	150
Garden salad/Caesar salad (before dressing)	150–350
Grilled chicken sandwich (6 oz)	280
Regular-sized hot dog with mustard and sauerkraut	300

SKIP	CALORIES
Nachos with cheese (many different sizes offered)	300–600
Chicken fingers/tenders (4, before dipping sauces)	400–600
Cracker Jack (whole bag, 980 g)	420
Large fries	500–575
Sausage pizza	350–500+

Box Seat Catering

Shea Stadium (New York Mets), Angel Stadium (Los Angeles Angels), Fenway Park (Boston Red Sox), Coors Field (Colorado Rockies), and McAfee Coliseum (Oakland Raiders) all have private box seat catering available through Aramark.

Menus for all locations have à la carte menu items like the following (each item serves 6 people):

PICK	CALORIES
Farmer's Market vegetable crudité	100–200
The season's best fruits and veggies	100–300
Fresh sushi platter	200–400
Jumbo shrimp cocktail	200–300
Chicken lettuce wraps	300–500

Yankee Stadium

Offers healthy options from Centerplate Catering for their Hall of Fame Suite guests.

PICK	CALORIES
Garden salad	100–200
Grilled chicken Caesar salad	200–400
Garden vegetable crudités	100–200
Fresh fruit and cheese display	200–300
Grilled fajitas	200–400
Grilled marinated chicken breast	150–350
Chilled roasted salmon	250–400
Sushi and sashimi platter	200–400
Grilled sliced beef tenderloin	200–400

Salad Bar Tips and Recipes

A salad bar can be an oasis of healthy eating or a fat trap. Many offices (as well as local delis and restaurants, of course) have extensive salad bars, and sometimes it's confusing to know how to fill your bowl. Here are the Wall Street steps to building a healthy, delicious salad:

- **CHOOSE THE DARKER GREENS. They're more nutritious. But if going dark deters you from having a salad at all, it is OK to pick a lighter lettuce.**

- **GO FOR THE SMALLER-SIZED GREENS. This will prevent you from adding too many ingredients.**

- **PICK A PROTEIN. Make sure it is grilled and not breaded. Best choices are: grilled chicken, roasted or fresh turkey, dry tuna (packed in water), shrimp, tofu (non-marinated), grilled steak (good for a change once a week), ham. Virgin Dieters or those who have over thirty pounds to lose can ask for a double portion of protein.**

- **PICK YOUR VEGGIES. Choose three non-starchy, non-marinated raw veggies. Choose from our list of veggies on the Wall Street Template (page 50).**

- **SKIP THE FOLLOWING: corn, beans, peas, chickpeas, roasted peppers, marinated mushrooms, caramelized onions, croutons, fried noodles, tortilla strips, sunflower seeds, dried fruit, candied nuts, potato/pasta salad, tuna/chicken salad made with mayo, full-fat dressing.**

- **VIRGIN DIETERS** or those who have more than thirty pounds to lose can add one small amount of optional fat such as olives, raw sliced almonds, sliced avocado, shredded cheese/mozzarella/ feta.

- **PICK A DRESSING.** Go for the light or low-fat balsamic if available. Use only one ladle. You can always add extra balsamic or red wine vinegar. If you don't like balsamic, you can go for another light or low-fat dressing, but really go easy on these, half a ladle, because the calories can still add up. You can also mix your own dressing of balsamic vinegar, olive oil (go easy on this), and Dijon mustard.

- **ADD A HEALTHY CRUNCH.** Crumble up two Fiber Rich crackers for a little fiber and crunch.

- **CHOP, CHOP!** The salads always taste best when you have them chopped up, so if that is a option, ask them to chop yours.

Wall Street Salad Bar Recipes

Tired of making the same old pile of greens in a bowl? Here are some Wall Street Salad Bar Recipes that will pique your taste buds. And of course they're healthy and low-cal.

NOTE:

In restaurants always ask for the light or low-fat dressing option and make sure you use only one ladle or half a ladle. You can always add balsamic or red wine vinegar for added flavor and minimal calories.

New Santa Fe Chicken Salad	Calories (279 total)
3 cups Romaine	25
3 oz grilled chicken breast	95
½ cup tomatoes	15
½ cup red peppers	12
½ cup onions	20
¼ cup red beans	45
¼ cup corn	40
2 T light balsamic vinaigrette	45

Asian Grilled Chicken Salad	Calories (335 total)
3 cups blend of spinach and Romaine	25
½ cup shredded carrots	22
½ oz slivered almonds	90
½ cup orange sections	40
½ cup sugar snap peas	13
3 oz grilled chicken breast	95
2 T low-fat Asian ginger vinaigrette	35
and add balsamic vinegar (2 T)	15

Chicken Caesar	Calories (276 total)
3 cups crispy Romaine lettuce	25
3 oz grilled chicken breast	95
2 T shaved Parmesan	50
2 high-fiber crackers (Fiber Rich) (broken up to act as croutons)	36
2 T light Caesar dressing	70

Beverly Hills Chef Salad	Calories (368 total with mozzarella, 320 total with imitation bacon bits)
3 cups iceberg and Romaine lettuce, mixed	25
2 slices deli turkey breast	40
2 slices deli ham	70
½ cup cucumber	8
½ cup tomato	15
1 oz mozzarella cheese	90
2 T imitation bacon bits	70
2 T nonfat honey Dijon	50

Miami Shrimp Salad	Calories (293 total)
3 cups Romaine lettuce	25
½ cup cucumber	8
½ cup tomato	15
¼ avocado	60
½ cup hearts of palm	20
3 oz grilled shrimp	85

Miami Shrimp Salad (continued)	Calories (293 total)
2 T low-fat cucumber dressing	80

Steakhouse Salad	Calories (260 total)
3 cups Romaine	25
3 oz grilled steak	155
1/2 cup onions	20
1/2 cup tomatoes	15
2 T light balsamic vinaigrette	45

Ten Vegetable Salad	Calories (285 total)
3 cups arugula	25
3 oz turkey	90
1/2 cup asparagus	22
1/2 cup green beans	15
1/2 cup cucumber	8
1/2 cup celery	10
1/2 cup tomato	15
1/2 cup broccoli	15
1/2 cup mushrooms	8
1/2 cup hearts of palm	20
1/2 cup cauliflower	12
2 T light balsamic vinaigrette	45

Tuna Niçoise Salad	Calories (302 total)
3 cups baby field greens	25
3 oz dry tuna (packed in water)	100
1/2 cup grape tomatoes	15
1/2 cup red onion	30
1/2 cup green beans	15
1/4 cup chopped egg	52
2 T olives	30
2 T low-fat Dijon mustard vinaigrette	35

High-dividend Chain Choices*

C hain restaurants are a fact of life. Many of us shun them because we think that they've got nothing on the menu that would be both tasty and healthy. (Of course some of us do the drive-through on the sly, but that's another matter!) The good news is that more of the chains are offering healthy choices. If you know what to pick, you can find a good low-calorie meal at a chain. This is important if you're traveling, in a rush, or ferrying the kids. Here is a good selection of national chains with their best and worst picks. You should know that all calorie data we've provided is from the chains themselves. We have to hope that they are correct. (Is it really possible that Panda Garden's Kung Pao Shrimp has only 240 calories? They say so.) You can always check their websites so you can find updates and further information if you're interested.

A few notes on choosing chain meals: We did list soup options, but individuals who are salt-sensitive must be aware of the sodium and should probably not choose a soup. If you are not salt-sensitive, you can always pick the soup and a veggie side and call it a meal. If the soup has

---

* Please note: not all choices are available in every outlet.

a Juicy Carb (like beans) in it and there is no other protein in the meal, then you do not need to count it as a Juicy Carb for the day. If you choose the soup and a main dish with protein, then the soup becomes your Juicy Carb. Where sandwiches or burgers are offered, you can always skip the bread (saving you a Juicy Carb) and request a house salad with dressing on the side (pick the lightest dressing available).

Applebee's

PICK	CALORIES
Onion soup	150
Grilled shrimp skewer salad	210
Cajun lime tilapia	310
Steak and portobellos	330
Italian chicken and portobello sandwich	360
Teriyaki Steak 'N Shrimp Skewers	370
Confetti Chicken	370

Note: **All items on special "Weight Watchers" menu.**

Arby's

PICK	CALORIES
Arby's Junior Roast Beef Sandwich (kids' menu)	272
Arby's Melt	302
Chicken Naturals Sandwich, chicken filet (grilled, no mayo)	310 (414 with mayo)
Martha's Vineyard Salad with raspberry vinaigrette	471 (277 without dressing)

SKIP	CALORIES
Classic Italian Toasted Sub	828
Ultimate BLT Sandwich	779

Au Bon Pain

BREAKFAST

PICK	CALORIES
Arugula and tomato frittata	290
Ham and cheddar frittata	320

SKIP	CALORIES
Chocolate chunk muffin	590
Plain bagel with egg, cheese, and bacon	560
Breakfast Prosciutto Sandwich	660

LUNCH

PICK	CALORIES
Southwest Vegetable Soup (medium)	100
Thai Chicken Salad	190
With fat-free raspberry vinaigrette (80)	270
Caesar salad	210
With fat-free raspberry vinaigrette (80)	290

SKIP	CALORIES
Shanghai Salad (with Asian sesame dressing)	980
Turkey melt	1030

Baja Fresh

PICK	CALORIES
Americano Soft Taco (chicken or shrimp)	230
Tortilla soup (without chicken)	270
Baja Ensalada: Charbroiled Chicken	310
With salsa verde (15)	325

SKIP	CALORIES
Charbroiled steak nachos	2120
Chicken fajitas with flour tortilla	1140

Bob Evans Family Restaurant

PICK	CALORIES
Vegetable beef soup (cup)	138
Plain salmon dinner	287
Salmon with garlic butter	326

SKIP	CALORIES
Cranberry pecan chicken salad	1142
Baby back ribs	1068

Burger King

BREAKFAST/LUNCH/DINNER

PICK	CALORIES
Side garden salad	15
With Ken's fat-free ranch dressing (60)	75
Croissan'wich Egg & Cheese (without the croissant)	150
Hamburger (without the bun)	160
Hamburger	290
TenderGrill Chicken Garden Salad (without dressing)	240
With Ken's Fat-Free Ranch Dressing (60)	300

KIDS' MENU

PICK	CALORIES
Flame-broiled Chicken Tenders (4-piece serving)	145
BK Fresh Apple Fries	35
BK Kids Meal (Chicken Tenders, Apple Fries, and low-fat milk)	305

SKIP	CALORIES
Triple Whopper sandwich	1130
BK Quad Stacker	1000

California Pizza Kitchen

They do not have calories listed on the company site. These are the best salad options with modifications:

- Grilled vegetable salad (no corn, no avocado, add grilled rosemary chicken or grilled shrimp, and request Dijon balsamic vinaigrette dressing on the side)

- Original chopped salad (no salami or cheese, and request Dijon balsamic vinaigrette on the side)

- Chinese chicken salad (skip the crispy wontons, skip the sesame seeds, and request Dijon balsamic vinaigrette on the side)

- Classic Caesar (order half size, add rosemary chicken breast or grilled shrimp, skip the croutons, and request Dijon balsamic vinaigrette on the side)

The Cheesecake Factory

A new line of salads, entitled Weight Management Salads, were added to the menu in January 2007. Each salad has less than 590 calories. Available in four varieties:

- Asian chicken salad
- Spicy chicken salad
- California salad
- Seafood salad

Chick-fil-A

PICK	CALORIES
Hearty Breast of Chicken Soup (small)	140
Chick-fil-A Chargrilled Chicken Garden Salad	180
With light Italian dressing (15)	195
Chick-fil-A Southwest Chargrilled Chicken Salad	240
Chick-fil-A Chargrilled Chicken Sandwich	270

SKIP	CALORIES
Chick-fil-A Chicken Caesar Cool Wrap	480
Chick-fil-A Chicken Deluxe Sandwich	420

Chili's/Chili's Too

Features a line of menu options called Guiltless Grill. (Available selection varies by location.)

PICK (FROM GUILTLESS GRILL)	CALORIES
Side steamed veggies with Parmesan cheese	60
Black bean burger patty only (no bun or topping)	200
With whole wheat bun (90)	290
Guiltless Salmon (follow $\frac{3}{4}$ Rule, cuts calories down)	480
Guiltless Chicken Sandwich (eat half the bread and save calories)	490
Grilled chicken Caesar salad (without croutons and balsamic vinaigrette dressing, calories not available)	

SKIP	CALORIES
Smoked turkey sandwich	930
Bacon burger	1080
Chicken Ranch Sandwich	1150
Awesome Blossom with Seasoned Sauce	2710

Così

BREAKFAST

PICK	CALORIES
Fruit salad	216

SKIP	CALORIES
Granola cereal	564
Apple crumb cake	540

PICK	CALORIES
Caesar salad	182
With fat-free balsamic vinaigrette (45)	227
Pollo E Pasta Soup Bowl	183
Shanghai Chicken Salad	221
With low-fat ginger soy dressing (74)	295
Brie and fruit plate	277
Build your own salad (greens, 1 protein, 3 non-starchy/non-marinated veggies, fat-free balsamic vinaigrette)	variable

SKIP	CALORIES
Roasted turkey and brie sandwich	772
Tuna cheddar melt	956

Dairy Queen

LUNCH/DINNER

PICK	CALORIES
Dairy Queen Grilled Chicken Salad	270
With fat-free Italian dressing (10)	280
With fat-free French dressing (40)	310
DQ Homestyle Burger	350
Dairy Queen Grilled Chicken Sandwich	350

SKIP	CALORIES
Dairy Queen Ultimate Burger	780
½ lb FlameThrower Grillburger	1030

Denny's

BREAKFAST

PICK	CALORIES
Quaker Oatmeal	100
Banana	110
Fit Fare: Veggie Egg Beater Omelet with English muffin	330

SKIP	CALORIES
Meat Lover's Breakfast	1230

LUNCH/DINNER

PICK	CALORIES
Chicken noodle soup	180
Fit Fare: Grilled Chicken Breast Dinner with sliced tomatoes, green beans	190
Fit Fare: Turkey Breast Salad	248
With low-calorie Italian dressing (15)	263
Fit Fare: Chicken Breast Salad	320
With low-calorie Italian Dressing (15)	335

SKIP	CALORIES
Jalapeño Burger with Fries	1480
Grilled chicken Alfredo entrée	1290

KFC

PICK	CALORIES
KFC Original Recipe chicken breast (no skin or breading) (360 with skin and breading)	140
Corn on the cob (3", 70 calories)	210
Honey BBQ Chicken Sandwich	280
Tender Roast Chicken Sandwich (without sauce)	300 (430 with sauce)
Oven Roasted Twister Sandwich (without sauce)	330 (470 with sauce)

SKIP	CALORIES
KFC Famous Bowls: mashed potatoes with gravy	740
Large Popcorn Chicken	550

Max & Erma's

Located in many U.S. airports, Max & Erma's only provides nutrition information for "No Guilt" menu offerings.

PICK (BEST "NO GUILT" CHOICES)	CALORIES
Baby Greens Salad (without breadstick)	119
With low-fat Tex Mex dressing (23)	142
With fat-free honey mustard (60)	179
Shrimp Stack Salad	322
Half Hula Bowl (with fat-free honey mustard dressing)	366
Fruit salad	54

SKIP	CALORIES
Black Bean Roll-Ups	577
Full Hula Bowl (without breadstick)	576

McDonald's

BREAKFAST

PICK	CALORIES
McDonald's Fruit 'n Yogurt Parfait (without granola)	130
Egg McMuffin (without the English Muffin)	160

SKIP	CALORIES
Deluxe Breakfast	1320
Hotcakes and sausage	780

PICK	CALORIES
Side salad	20
With low-fat balsamic vinaigrette (40)	60
McDonald's Hamburger (without the bun)	90
Fruit and walnut salad (snack size)	210
Caesar salad with grilled chicken	220
With low-fat balsamic vinaigrette (40)	260
McDonald's Hamburger	250
Honey Mustard Snack Wrap (grilled chicken)	260
Asian Salad with Grilled Chicken	300
With low-fat balsamic vinaigrette (40)	340

SKIP	CALORIES
Double Quarter Pounder with Cheese	740
With medium French fries (380)	1120
Premium Crispy Chicken Club Sandwich	660

Olive Garden

Olive Garden doesn't provide nutrition information for main menu items but does feature a healthier line called Garden Fare. Always hit the salad bar with our recommended salad bar picks.

PICK (FROM GARDEN FARE)	CALORIES
Minestrone soup	164
Venetian Apricot Chicken	328

SKIP	CALORIES
Capellini Pomodoro (dinner entrée)	644
Shrimp Primavera (dinner entrée)	706

Panda Express

PICK	CALORIES
Mixed Veggies	70
Veggie Spring Roll (1 piece)	80
Hot and Sour Soup	110
Mushroom Chicken	130
Tangy Shrimp	150
Broccoli Beef	150
Chicken Breast with String Beans	160
Eggplant and Tofu in Garlic Sauce	180
Black Pepper Chicken	200
Kung Pao Shrimp	240
Mandarin Chicken	250

SKIP	CALORIES
Orange Chicken	500
BBQ Pork	440

Note: All chicken, beef, and shrimp dishes listed are served as 5.5-oz portions. Steamed rice (8-oz portion) is 380 calories. Skip rice, as sauce in all dishes will count as Juicy Carb.

Panera Bread

PICK	CALORIES
French onion soup (no cheese or croutons, 8 oz)	80
Low-fat chicken noodle soup (8 oz)	100
Low-fat vegetarian black bean soup (8 oz)	160
Grilled salmon salad (half portion)	170
Asian sesame salad (half portion)	220
Grilled chicken Caesar salad (half portion)	280
Strawberry poppyseed and chicken salad (full)	310
Note: All salads are estimated without dressing.	
Fat-free poppyseed dressing (2 oz)	30
Fat-free raspberry dressing (2 oz)	50
Smoked turkey on sourdough sandwich (half portion)	230
Half Chicken Pomodoro hot panini on French (half portion)	280
Fresh fruit cup (small)	70

SKIP	CALORIES
Italian Combo Sandwich (full portion)	1100
Tuna salad on whole grain	840

PF Chang's

PICK	CALORIES
Shanghai Cucumbers	120
Buddha's Feast, steamed	200
Cantonese Shrimp	330
Steamed shrimp dumpling appetizer	330

SKIP	CALORIES
Beef with broccoli dinner	1120
Lo Mein vegetable dinner	1340

Pizza Hut

PICK	CALORIES
1 slice 14" Fit n' Delicious Pizza (6 different varieties)	230 (or less, per slice)
2 slices 12" Fit n' Delicious Pizza	
Green pepper, red onion, diced red tomato	300
Ham and pineapple	320
Diced chicken, mushroom, and jalapeño	320

SKIP	CALORIES
2 slices 12" Medium Pan Meat Lover's Pizza	740
6" Personal Pan Pepperoni Pizza	640

Popeyes Chicken & Biscuits

PICK THE BREAST PLUS EITHER THE THIGH, WING, OR LEG, AND A SIDE OF GREEN BEANS.	CALORIES
Mild or spicy chicken breast (skinless, and breading removed)	120
Mild or spicy chicken thigh (skinless, and breading removed)	80
Mild or spicy chicken wing (skinless and breading removed)	40
Mild or spicy chicken leg (skinless and breading removed)	50
Green beans side	70

SKIP	CALORIES
Deluxe Sandwich with mayo	630
Chicken and Sausage Jambalaya	660

Red Lobster

Red Lobster features a healthier line of food options called LightHouse. (Availability varies by location.)

PICK	CALORIES
Grilled jumbo shrimp dinner	142
Live Maine lobster (1¼ lbs)	145 (without butter)
Broiled flounder dinner	240
Grilled chicken breast	315
Tilapia (full portion)	346

SKIP	CALORIES
Atlantic salmon (full portion)	578
Wild rice pilaf side dish	205

Ruby Tuesday's

All recommended items are from the Smart Eating line of options.

PICK	CALORIES
Tossed Caesar salad	175
With lite ranch dressing (55)	230
7-oz sirloin steak (no sides)	206
White bean chicken chili	257
Grilled chicken (no sides)	295
Creole catch (tilapia)	312
Grilled chicken salad	380
Premium baby green beans (lowest caloric side to add)	85

SKIP	CALORIES
Ruby's Classic Burger	1013
Chicken and Broccoli Penne	1646

7-Eleven

BREAKFAST

PICK	CALORIES
Instant oatmeal (maple brown sugar)	210
Eggs Anytime (two hard-boiled)	140
Crystal Light slurpee (ordered anytime)	64

SKIP	CALORIES
Sausage, egg, cheese biscuit	500
Banana nut muffin	660

Starbucks

(Available in participating stores, offerings vary regionally.)

BREAKFAST

PICK	CALORIES
Any version of non- or low-fat yogurt	60–160
Any breakfast wrap or sandwich under 300 calories	200–300
Reduced-fat turkey bacon, egg, and reduced-fat white cheddar sandwich	350

SKIP	CALORIES
Classic Sausage, Egg & Cheddar	470
Scones (various flavors)	480–500
Regular muffins (not low/reduced fat)	420–500

LUNCH

PICK	CALORIES
Low-fat turkey and artichoke sandwich	190
Turkey and Swiss sandwich (no condiments)	280
Tomato Mozzarella Insalata	280
Very Veggie Crunch Wrap	310
Asian-style layered salad	310
Vegetable Vinaigrette	310
Fiesta Salad	320
Fruit and cheese plate	370

SKIP	CALORIES
Chicken cheddar club with bacon	550
Egg salad on multigrain	470
Garden tuna salad wrap	460

Subway

Trend: Subway now has a line of healthy meals called Subway Fresh Fit Meals, which include a side of fruit (35 calories for an apple slice packet) and a bottle of water. Calorie info below is for salad/sandwich only.

PICK	CALORIES
Jared (low-fat) Salads: ham, roast beef, club, turkey breast, or Veggie Delite	150 (or less)
Any above salad with fat-free Italian dressing (35)	185 (or less)
6" Jared (low-fat) Sandwiches:	
Veggie Delite	230
Turkey breast	280
Ham	290
Roast beef	290
Oven-roasted chicken breast	310

Note: These do not include dressing or sauces. Suggest mustard or vinegar to keep calories low.

SKIP	CALORIES
6" Double Meatball Marinara Sub	860
6" Double Subway Steak and Cheese Sub	540

Taco Bell

Menu includes Fresco Style items, which contain 10 g of fat or less.

PICK	CALORIES
Grilled Steak Soft Taco ("Fresco Style")	160
Ranchero Chicken Soft Taco ("Fresco Style")	170
Taco Bell Beef Soft Taco Supreme ("Fresco Style")	190
Taco Bell Enchirito, Beef ("Fresco Style")	230
Taco Bell Gordita Baja Chicken	320

SKIP	CALORIES
Chicken Fiesta Taco Salad	800
Taco Bell "Grilled Stuft" Chicken Burrito	640

T.G.I. Friday's

Friday's does not publish nutrition information for their main menu. The menu does include a few options that they consider to be healthier. For example:

LOW-FAT OPTIONS (EACH HAS ABOUT 10G FAT AND 500 CALORIES)
- **Dragonfire Chicken**
- **Zen Chicken Pot Stickers (the dumpling counts as a Juicy Carb for the day)**

LOW-CARB OPTIONS (ALL AVOID THE JUICY CARB BUT BECAUSE OF FAT CONTENT WILL BE HIGHER IN CALORIES)
- **Sizzling Chicken & Vegetables (eat only 25% of the cheese)**
- **Shrimp Key West**

There are salad options not listed in the low-fat/low-carb section; however, you need to make modifications to lower the calories and Juicy Carbs. Follow the ¾ Rule to cut additional calories. Here are the best picks:

- **Strawberry Fields salad with chicken (no pecans and dressing on the side)**
- **Caesar salad with cedar-seared salmon (no croutons, and request balsamic vinaigrette on the side)**
- **Bistro sirloin salad (no corn; request balsamic vinaigrette on the side)**

Also, Friday's features six new entrées for the new Right Portion, Right Price ($6.99–$8.99) menu. However, only two of the offerings, Dragonfire Chicken and Shrimp Key West, are Wall Street Diet approved.

Wendy's

PICK	CALORIES
Wendy's Mandarin Chicken Salad (without noodles or almonds)	170
With fat-free French dressing (70)	240
Small chili	220
Wendy's Jr. Hamburger	280
Wendy's Grilled Chicken Sandwich	310

SKIP	CALORIES
Southwest Taco Salad with Ancho Chipotle Ranch Dressing	680
Wendy's Old Fashioned Burgers: ½ lb Double with Cheese	700

Wall Street Restaurant Menu Survival Guide

UNIVERSAL RESTAURANT TIPS

- Have two Fiber Rich crackers and drink 8 ounces of water before you go out to eat. This will curb your appetite.

- Before you arrive, decide which of the following you want: bread, two glasses of wine, or a shared dessert.

- Wear clothing that is tight around the waist.

- Do not eat off anyone else's plate.

- Follow the 3/4 Rule.

- Order two appetizers instead of an entrée where available and appealing.

- Put your fork/knife down at least three times and take your time.

- Choose grilled, roasted, or baked foods.

- Have your water glass filled three times.

AMERICAN

- Appetizer: salad with shaved Parmesan, grilled calamari, or tuna tartare

- Entrée: whole roasted fish or other grilled/roasted lean protein (veal, lamb, or poultry)

- Sides: sautéed vegetable and roasted/baked potatoes

- Dessert: poached pear, fruit plate, sorbet (not coconut), or decaf skim cappuccino/herbal tea

Choose one of the following:

- Egg-white omelet with 1 slice cheese and 2 veggies, salad, no home fries, and optional side of fruit salad or 2 slices Canadian bacon
- Oatmeal made with water, and small fruit salad
- 2 poached eggs with lettuce and tomato and fruit salad
- Eggs Benedict (no hollandaise sauce, English muffin=Juicy Carb)
- Eggs Florentine (no hollandaise sauce; skip muffin, extra spinach)

CHINESE

- Start with hot and sour or egg drop soup, small size (only for those who are not salt-sensitive).
- Best option is any dish with a steamed protein and veggies.
- Ask for the sauce on the side and for no sugar, cornstarch, or MSG.
- Pick either brown rice or a fist-sized portion of either steamed vegetable or shrimp dumplings and count as your Juicy Carb.
- Another entrée option is moo shoo chicken, steamed. Add half of the container of hoisen sauce and light soy sauce.
- Avoid sweet-and-sour choices; they're often deep-fried; avoid egg rolls and crunchy noodles.
- Eat all meals with chopsticks to help slow you down.

FRENCH BISTRO

- Appetizer: arugula and shaved Parmesan, mixed green salad with goat cheese, oysters on the half shell, shrimp cocktail, or French onion soup, no bread, no cheese (not for salt-sensitive)
- Entrée: grilled fish and veggies, or moules (mussels) in white wine/garlic broth (no frites, ask for salad instead), or steak with salad (no frites)
- Can also do two appetizers—salad and either oysters, shrimp cocktail, moules, or tuna tartare

GREEK/MEDITERRANEAN

- Appetizer: tomato/cucumber salad
- One Juicy Carb: hummus with 1/4 pita or 1 fist of rice with meal
- Entrée: grilled fish or grilled chicken/shrimp kabob

INDIAN

- Appetizer: tandoori vegetables
- Entrée: chicken tikka (not tikka masala) or chicken/shrimp tandoori
- Remember that $\frac{1}{2}$ roti bread, 1 fist rice or 2 pappadum = Juicy Carb.

ITALIAN

- Appetizer: mixed green salad and/or mussels
- Entrée: grilled fish (or another protein grilled) of the day plus a side order of any green vegetable (steamed if possible) or shrimp marinara (sauce is Juicy Carb), or chicken scarpariello (sauce is Juicy Carb)
- Avoid: cream sauces, anything "alfredo," pasta dishes

JAPANESE

- To start: miso soup (good option for those who are not salt-sensitive) or mixed green salad with half ginger dressing or seaweed salad
- Next: chicken/salmon teriyaki with double steamed veggies (no rice, sauce is Juicy Carb) or maki roll (6 pieces = Juicy Carb) plus 4 pieces sashimi and side order oshitashi (spinach) or 8 pieces sashimi with side of oshitashi or one cucumber roll with 4 pieces sashimi and side order of oshitashi
- Avoid: tempura, spider, dynamite, spicy rolls, and eel
- Avoid dishes described as Agemono or tempura, both of which are deep fried.
- Steer clear of sushi rolls made with cream cheese and too much avocado.
- Always request lite soy sauce and add wasabi (those who are salt-sensitive should use lemon only).
- Eat with chopsticks to help slow you down.

MEXICAN

- Choose your one Juicy Carb before you arrive (e.g., chips with salsa, place handful of chips on side plate and no additional chips, or a fist-sized portion of rice or beans).
- Always ask for sliced jicama instead of chips.
- For your entrée choose the grilled chicken or shrimp fajita with sautéed veggies (skip the guacamole and sour cream, and no margaritas, choose light beer instead).

PIZZA

- Order one slice of thin-crust with vegetables (counts as one Juicy Carb) and one large salad.

- Virgin Dieters or those who need to lose more than thirty pounds can have two slices.

STEAK HOUSE

- Choose grilled entrées.

- Order the smallest size steak.

- Filet mignon is a good lean choice that's a reasonable size.

- Skip the creamed spinach and choose steamed or sautéed vegetables.

- Skip the baked potato and choose double vegetables.

- Choose a tossed salad with light dressing and skip coleslaw.

THAI

- Appetizer: tom yum soup (chicken or shrimp)

- Entrée: pick appetizer combinations, either chicken saté (no peanut sauce), Thai salad, and tom yum soup, or soup plus Thai beef or shrimp salad

- Entrée: soup to start and share shrimp or chicken in chili basil sauce, no rice (the sauce counts as a Juicy Carb)

Movie Theater
Picks and Skips

M ovie theaters are hotbeds of mindless eating. But sometimes it's hard to watch a film without munching. So follow my guidelines and your butt won't become a double feature!

FIRST PICK	CALORIES
17 grapes	60
Polly-O string cheese	80
2 Babybel Light	100
Orville Redenbacher Smart Pop Mini Bag	100
Ziploc of fresh strawberries (2 cups)	100
Glenny's Soy Crisps (1.3-oz bag)	140
Luna or any bar under 200	200 (or less)

Or bring any Fun Snack in Shopping List (pages 311–312). Skip the Fun Snack between lunch and dinner and save for the movie.

SECOND PICK	CALORIES
Child-sized bag of popcorn (no added butter)	280–300

Even a small popcorn without butter will set you back 400 calories. Unless there is a child-sized bag available, avoid the popcorn altogether. Keep in mind when fighting off temptation that a large popcorn with butter packs in an entire day's worth of calories!

SKIP	CALORIES
Small popcorn (no added butter)	400
Small popcorn (with butter)	580
Medium popcorn (no added butter)	900
Medium popcorn (with butter)	1325
Large popcorn (plain)	1150
Large popcorn (with butter)	1650

Candy at the movie theater typically comes in a king-sized package, so even lower-fat sweets like Twizzlers, Gummi Bears, and Junior Mints are caloric disasters! Higher-fat items like Reese's Pieces will set you back over 1000 calories!

SKIP	CALORIES
Mike and Ike (3-oz box)	320
Junior Mints (3-oz box)	360
Milk Duds (3-oz box)	370
Gummi Bears (3.5-oz bag)	390
Raisinets (3.5-oz bag)	400
Starburst (4.4 oz)	480
Goobers (3.5-oz box)	500
Twizzlers (6-oz bag)	570
M&M's (5.3-oz bag)	750
Skittles (6.5-oz bag)	765
Peanut M&M's (5.3-oz bag)	790
Dots (9.2-oz box)	850
Reese's Pieces (8-oz bag)	1160

- Bring or buy bottled water.

- Have a balanced meal at home or out before the movie (pick later movie time).

- Don't start eating the snack you have chosen until the movie starts.

National and International Airport Terminal Food Options

H ere is a selection of the best food options at the busiest domestic airport terminals as well as London and Hong Kong. The calorie information is directly from the restaurants themselves and we have to rely on their accuracy. In many instances, we've provided websites that you can access for more detailed or up-to-date information on these restaurants. For more detailed recommendations on the best options at the chain restaurants, see "High-dividend Chain Choices," page 237.

Hudson News, located at almost every airport in the nation, is listed first and separately. Otherwise the airports are listed in alphabetical order by city, national terminals first.

Hudson News

Best bet at Hudson News is to choose a bar (see below), bottled water, a pack of sugar-free gum, and some reading material. All other food choices should be skipped. See note below.

PICK	CALORIES
Soy Joy bar	130–140
Nature Valley trail mix bar	140
Nature Valley granola bar (2-bar pack)	180
South Beach meal replacement bar	210
Balance Gold, caramel nut blast	210
Balance bar, almond brownie or honey peanut	200
PowerBar Harvest, peanut butter chocolate chip	240
PowerBar Harvest, strawberry crunch	240
PowerBar Harvest, double chocolate crisp	250

SKIP	CALORIES (WHOLE BAG)
Fig Newtons	200
Snyder's Olde Tyme Pretzels	240
Barnum's Animal Crackers	240
Keebler Elfin Crackers	260
Jack Link's beef jerky (teriyaki flavor)	280
Häagen-Dazs ice cream bar	320
Peanut M&M's (3.27-oz bag)	480
Snickers (king-sized bar)	541
Goldfish crackers (6.6-oz bag)	840
Simply Almonds & Raisins	678
Peanuts (3.5-oz bag)	510

Skip These Nut and Dried Fruit Options

(Based on Snack Club Brand, check out the calories!)

SNACK	SERVING SIZE	CALS/ SERVING	SERVINGS/ BAG	TOTAL CALS/ BAG
Raw trail mix	⅓ c	131	8	1048
Yogurt nut mix	¼ c	124	8	992
Cranberry trail mix	⅓ c	130	7	910
Salted soy beans	3 T or ⅓ c	140	7	980
Raw almonds	22 pc	181	3	543

Note: There are many different nut/fruit options and the brands may vary by location. These products are definitely a diet trap because they all say "no cholesterol/no preservatives." You'd think they would be healthy, particularly with names of foods in the package like yogurt, raw, cranberry, soy beans . . . Most people associate these choices with nutritious foods, so beware!

Hartsfield-Jackson Atlanta International Airport

1. Burger King (Concourses A, D, T)
See p. 289 for top recommendations.

2. Chick-fil-A (Concourse A)

PICK	CALORIES
Hearty Breast of Chicken Soup (small)	140
Chick-fil-A Chargrilled Chicken Garden Salad	180
With light Italian dressing (15)	195
Chick-fil-A Southwest Chargrilled Chicken Salad	240
Chick-fil-A Chargrilled Chicken Sandwich	270

SKIP	CALORIES
Chick-fil-A Chicken Caesar Cool Wrap	480
Chick-fil-A Chicken Deluxe Sandwich	420

3. Chili's Too/To Go (Concourses A, D)
See pp. 289–90 for top recommendations.

4. Great Wraps (Concourse A)
Menu lets consumers "build their own" so nutrition info is broken out by ingredients.

PICK (INSTRUCTIONS FOR BUILDING YOUR WRAP)	CALORIES
1 meat	70–90
1 bread	220
Plain mustard	0
Shredded lettuce	0
2–3 vegetables	30 max
Total: 320-calorie sandwich	

MEAT PICKS	CALORIES
2 oz pork	73
3.5 oz chicken	78
3.5 oz turkey	80
2 oz ham	80
4 oz large chicken tenderloin	90

VEGGIE PICKS	CALORIES
2 oz shredded lettuce	0
1 oz chopped cucumber	2.5
1 oz green pepper	4
1 oz garlic mushrooms	5
2 oz spinach	5
1 oz chopped pepperoncini	5
2 oz chopped tomatoes	10
2 oz Romaine	10
1 oz chopped onion	10

BREAD PICKS	CALORIES
7" pita	220

DRESSING PICKS	CALORIES
1 oz balsamic vinaigrette	60

MEAT SKIPS	CALORIES
3.5-oz gyro	350
3.5 oz tuna	105
4 oz steak	110
All cheese options	160–220

VEGGIE SKIPS	CALORIES
3 oz portobello mushrooms	81
1 oz black olives	60

BREAD SKIPS	CALORIES
12" flour tortilla	320
12" spinach tortilla	290
12" tomato-basil tort	320

DRESSING SKIPS	CALORIES
2 oz Caesar	300
2 oz honey mustard	280
2 oz lite ranch	200
1 oz Cuban sauce	170

5. Houlihan's (Concourse A, Atrium)
(calories not provided by company)

PICK

Lettuce wraps

Grilled rosemary chicken (ask to be served
without Red Bliss Mashed Potatoes)

Atlantic salmon, 8 oz (share or eat only half, order
simply prepared option and skip mashed potatoes)

Grilled shrimp (skip mayo dipping sauce and add side salad)

Ahi tuna salad (ask to omit cashews and crispy wonton strips)

SKIP

Creamy Gorgonzola Burger

Stuffed potato skins

Chipotle Chicken Nachos

Baby back BBQ ribs

Chicken finger platter (with fries)

Ranchhouse Steak Salad

(Again, menu items seem high in calories just by
looking—may not want to include.)

6. Manchu Wok (Concourse A, Atrium)
See p. 291 for top recommendations.

7. Starbucks (Concourses A, B, E, T)
See p. 294 for top recommendations.

8. McDonald's (Concourse E)
See p. 292 for top recommendations.

9. Qdoba Mexican Grill (Concourse E)

PICK	CALORIES
Tortilla Soup	150
Grilled Veggie Naked Taco Salad	240
Naked Chicken Taco Salad	310

SKIP	CALORIES
Fajita Ranchera Naked Burrito	530
Chicken Mexican Gumbo	710
Grilled Vegetable Burrito	790

10. Au Bon Pain (Concourse B)
See pp. 288–89 for top recommendations.

Boston Logan International Airport

1. Fresh City (Terminal A)

PICK	CALORIES
Farmer's Carrot Broccoli Soup	123
Fresh City Chicken Soup	136
All-American Turkey (with mustard) on low-carb tortilla	251
Chicken Stir Fry (ask for no rice and ½ sauce)	287
Mandarin Sesame Chicken Salad (no wonton strips)	321

SKIP	CALORIES
Sirloin Steak Burrito	782
Buffalo Bleu Wrap	677

2. Wendy's (Terminal A)
See p. 295 for top recommendations.

3. Au Bon Pain (Terminals A, B, C, E)
See pp. 288–89 for top recommendations.

4. Starbucks (Terminals A, B, C)
See p. 294 for top recommendations.

5. McDonald's (Terminals B, E)
See p. 292 for top recommendations.

6. Asian TOO (Terminal B)

(calories not provided by company)

PICK

Sushi: tuna roll or vegetable roll with a side of mixed vegetables or soup of the day

Sushi Nigiri Platter (1 piece each of tuna, salmon, shrimp, and eel)

SKIP

Cheesy Crabby Wontons

Orange Chicken

General Tso's Chicken

7. Così (Terminal B)

See p. 290 for top recommendations

8. KnowFat! Café (Terminal B, expected to be completed by spring 2008)

The following is from the Regular Menu.

PICK	CALORIES
Three Bean Chili Bowl	210
All White Meat Chicken Chili Bowl	274
Spring Mix Tuna Salad	293
Southwestern Steak Salad	327
Steamed Chicken Tenderloins with steamed broccoli and brown rice (small)	339
California Tuna Salad Wrap (small)	341
Fire-Roasted Turkey Wrap (small)	347

SKIP	CALORIES
Fajita Burrito with chicken (regular)	682
Grilled Veggie Melt	606

9. Legal Sea Foods (Terminal B)

(calories not provided by company)

PICK

Raw oysters (available from 1 oyster to a dozen)

Jumbo shrimp cocktail

Mixed field greens topped with Maine crabmeat (ask for balsamic vinaigrette on the side)

Blackened raw tuna sashimi

Fried calamari

Fish and chips

10. Uno Chicago Grill (Terminal C)

PICK	CALORIES
Veggie Soup	120
Tuscan Pesto Minestrone Soup	150
Chicken Lettuce Wraps	200
Cuban Black Bean and Lentil Soup	220
Grilled mahi-mahi with mango salsa	220
BBQ Grilled Shrimp	250
House salad with grilled chicken	250 (with fat)
Free vinaigrette (30)	280
7-oz. filet mignon	290
Greek salad	300
With fat-free vinaigrette (30)	330

SKIP	CALORIES
Tuscan Chicken Penne	1220
Turkey bacon and Swiss sandwich	1100

Chicago O'Hare International Airport

1. Manchu Wok (Terminals 1, 3)
See p. 291 for top recommendations.

2. McDonald's (Terminals 1, 2, 3, 5)
See p. 292 for top recommendations.

3. Chili's (Terminals 1, 2, 3)
See pp. 289–290 for top recommendations.

4. Corner Bakery (Terminals 1, 3)

PICK	CALORIES
Cucumber Tomato Salad	60
Fruit Medley Salad	90
Zesty Chicken Tortilla Soup (10 oz)	230
Roasted Tomato Basil Soup (15 oz)	240
Mom's Chicken Noodle Soup (15 oz)	250
Black Bean Soup (10 oz)	260

SKIP	CALORIES
Loaded Baked Potato Soup (15 oz)	650
Chicken Carbonara	1300
Harvest Salad	860

5. Panda Express (Terminals 1, 3)

See p. 293 for top recommendations.

6. Salad Works (Terminal 1)

(calories not provided by company)

For all salads ask for lite balsamic with sundried tomato or lite ranch dressing.

PICK

Garden Salad with Grilled Chicken or Shrimp

Shrimp Caesar Salad with lite balsamic dressing, no Caesar

Make Your Own Salad: follow Salad Bar Guidelines

Tuscan Bean Minestrone Soup

Vegetarian Vegetable Soup

SKIP

Buffalo Chicken Wrap

New England Clam Chowder

7. Berghoff Café (Terminal 1)

(calories not provided by company)

PICK

Asian salad with chicken (request no wontons, dressing on the side)

Pear salad with grilled chicken (request no candied walnuts, dressing on the side)

Caesar salad (request no wontons, dressing on the side)

SKIP

Weiner Schnitzel

Italian Combo Sandwich

8. O'Brian's Pub (Terminal 3)

(calories not provided by company)

PICK

Oysters on the half shell

Gulf shrimp cocktail

Grilled rosemary chicken with vegetables (carb smart)

Caesar salad with grilled chicken (request balsamic vinaigrette on the side)

O'Brian's Special Salad (artichoke hearts, hearts of palm, onion, egg, and tomato; request balsamic vinaigrette on the side)

Chicken sandwich (request whole wheat bread, no mayo)

SKIP

Steak sandwich

Shepherd's pie

9. Burrito Beach (Terminal 3)

(calories not provided by company)

PICK

Grilled Veggie "Beach Bowl"

Grilled Marinated Chicken "Beach Bowl"

Soft flour tacos: grilled chicken or grilled veggie (no cheese)

SKIP

Buffalo chicken burrito

Ground beef burrito

Cleveland Hopkins International Airport

1. Burger King (Concourse C, Food Court)

See p. 289 for top recommendations.

2. Manchu Wok (Food Court)

See p. 291 for top recommendations.

3. Starbucks (Plaza, Concourse D, Main Ticketing Area)

See p. 294 for top recommendations.

4. Max & Erma's (Concourses B, C)

See pp. 291–92 for top recommendations.

5. Great Lakes Brewing Co. (Concourse A)

(calories not provided by company)

House salad with low-fat or light dressing or vinaigrette

Market Avenue Salad with Grilled Chicken with low-fat or light dressing or vinaigrette

Dortmunder Chicken Sandwich (recommend skipping the bun; ask for mustard instead of mayo and order side salad, no fries)

Grilled salmon, served with green beans, risotto, and a garnish of julienned carrots, zucchini, and squash (order without risotto)

SKIP

Catfish Sandwich (fried and served with fries)

Chicken Salad Croissant

Pepperoni and Sausage Pizza

6. Jody Maroni's (Concourse D)

PICK	CALORIES
Smoked chicken apple sausage	200
Tequila chicken sausage	200
Smoked chicken andouille sausage	200
Hot Italian sausage	260
Mild bratwurst	260

SKIP

(calories not provided by company)

Special meals with regular fries and soda

Jumbo-sized hot dog

Coney Island hot dog (with chili and cheddar cheese)

Dallas/Fort Worth International Airport

1. McDonald's (Terminals A, B, C, D, E)
See p. 292 for top recommendations.

2. Manchu Wok (Terminals A, C, D, E)
See p. 291 for top recommendations.

3. Starbucks Coffee (Terminals A, B, C, D, E)
See p. 294 for top recommendations.

4. Wendy's (Terminal C)
See p. 295 for top recommendations.

5. Dickey's BBQ (Terminal C)

PICK	CALORIES
Fresh fruit salad	60
Green beans	70
Cucumber salad	110
Stir-fried broccoli	120
Caesar salad	130
With 2 oz olive vinaigrette (15)	145
Pork tenderloin	250
Chicken breast	280

SKIP	CALORIES
Macaroni and cheese	590
Beef ribs	590

6. Champps Grill & Bar (Terminal D)
(calories not provided by company)

PICK

Bowl of soup and side salad (choose a side garden salad and French onion soup; request no crostini or cheese)

Grilled salmon (request no pecan brown butter sauce or mashed potatoes)

Balsamic Glazed Chicken (chicken marinated in balsamic vinaigrette and served with fresh vegetables)

Pan Pacific Chicken Salad (marinated chicken with mixed greens, crispy wonton strips, red onions, carrots, red peppers, bamboo shoots, water chestnuts, mandarin oranges, and spicy peanuts, with your choice of Thai peanut or orange ginger dressing) (ask for orange ginger dressing on the side and request no crispy wonton strips, no mandarin oranges, and no spicy peanuts)

SKIP

Half rack baby back ribs

Chicken and broccoli penne

7. Einstein Bros. Bagels (Terminal D)

PICK	CALORIES
Chicken Noodle Soup Bowl	160
Thai Soup Bowl	170
Naked Eggs, plain	270
Naked Eggs, Black Forest ham	320
Roasted turkey and swiss on artisan wheat (request no swiss cheese or creamy mustard spread)	320
Turkey Chili Bowl	330
Naked Eggs, sausage	340

SKIP	CALORIES
Vegetable Breakfast Panini	750
Bros. Bistro Salad	810

8. Popeyes Chicken & Biscuits (Terminal D)
See p. 293 for top recommendations.

9. 360 Gourmet Burrito (Terminal D)

PICK	CALORIES
Cajun Prawns Salad	290
Mediterranean Prawns Salad	290
Classic 360 Smoked Tofu Salad	319
Teriyaki Steak Salad	323
Teriyaki Chicken Breast Salad	346

SKIP	CALORIES
Cajun Steak Quesadilla	914
Thai Chicken Wrap	904
Cajun Steak Wrap	855
360 Gourmet Burrito (original)	610

10. Burger King (Terminal E)
See p. 289 for top recommendations.

Denver International Airport

1. Burger King (Terminal Level 6)

See p. 289 for top recommendations.

2. Chef Jimmy's Bistro & Spirits (Concourse A)

(calories not provided by company)

PICK

Original Chicken Sandwich without mayo (ask for no butter on roll)

Grilled Mahi-Mahi Platter, no fries (ask for baked potato or grilled vegetables instead)

Mediterranean Grilled Shrimp with side selection of grilled vegetables (no mashed potatoes or fries)

Bistro Salad (order without cheese, add grilled chicken)

3. McDonald's (Concourses A, B, C)

See p. 292 for top recommendations.

4. Panda Express (Concourse A, Terminal Level 6)

See p. 293 for top recommendations.

5. Heidi's Brooklyn Deli (Concourse B-Regional Jet Facility)

(calories not provided by company)

PICK

Ham sandwich (no cheese) with mustard on light rye

Veggie sandwich (replace cream cheese with mustard) on light rye

Heidi's Combo (½ sandwich with soup) (suggest broth-based soup and ham or turkey sandwich with mustard on light rye)

Cajun Turkey Sandwich with avocado on light rye (skip avocado to save calories)

SKIP

Bronx Bomber (pastrami and egg salad on rye)

Transplanted New Yorker Sandwich

Chicken salad sandwich

Hell's Kitchen Sandwich (egg salad, bacon, swiss, etc.)

6. Airmeals (Concourse C)

(calories not provided by company)

PICK

Fruit salad (different sizes are available)

Garden salad

Chef salad (recommend omitting cheese and selecting low-fat, fat-free or vinaigrette dressing)

Turkey sandwich with cheese on wheat bread (recommend removing cheese)*

Ham sandwich with cheese on wheat bread (recommend removing cheese)*

Selection of yogurts is available

7. KFC

PICK	CALORIES
KFC Original Recipe Chicken Breast (no skin or breading)	140 (360 with skin and breading)
Honey BBQ Chicken Sandwich	280
Tender Roast Chicken Sandwich (without sauce)	300 (430 with sauce)
Oven Roasted Twister Sandwich (without sauce)	330 (470 with sauce)

SKIP	CALORIES
KFC Famous Bowls: mashed potatoes with gravy	740
Large Popcorn Chicken	550

Detroit Metro Airport

Detroit Airport is made up of three main terminals: McNamara, Smith, and Berry.

MCNAMARA TERMINAL DINING

1. Burger King (Central Link Area)

See p. 289 for top recommendations.

2. Chili's (Gate A36)

See pp. 289–90 for top recommendations.

3. Max & Erma's (Gate A30)

See pp. 291–92 for top recommendations.

---

* These sandwiches are sold with mayo on the side.

4. McDonald's (Gate A36)

See p. 292 for top recommendations.

5. Rio Wraps (Gate A60)

(calories not provided by company)

PICK

Turkey with a Twist Sandwich (order without cheese and request low-fat or fat-free dressing)

Veggie Wrap, without guacamole (order on a low-carb garden vegetable wrap or a mini whole wheat wrap)

Rio Salad with grilled chicken (order without cheese)

6. Waterworks Bar & Grill (Gate A1)

(calories not provided by company)

PICK

Salads made to order (follow salad bar guidelines, p. 233)

Chicken and/or vegetable stir-fry

Sandwiches made to order (follow deli guidelines, pp. 225–26)

7. Taco Bell (Gate A74)

PICK	CALORIES
Grilled Steak Soft Taco ("Fresco Style")	160
Ranchero Chicken Soft Taco ("Fresco Style")	170
Taco Bell Beef Soft Taco Supreme ("Fresco Style")	190
Taco Bell Enchirito, Beef ("Fresco Style")	230

SKIP	CALORIES
Chicken Fiesta Taco Salad	800
Taco Bell "Grilled Stuft" Chicken Burrito	640

Miami International Airport

1. Au Bon Pain (Concourses A, G)

See pp. 288–89 for top recommendations.

2. Starbucks (Most concourses)

See p. 294 for top recommendations.

3. Chili's To Go and Snack Bar (Concourses E, F, and G)

See pp. 289–90 for top recommendations.

4. Manchu Wok (Concourse D)

See p. 291 for top recommendations.

5. Top of the Port Restaurant

This restaurant is buffet style, and the menu changes daily. There is always a salad bar, and there are always fresh, healthy soups available.

6. California Pizza Kitchen

See p. 289 for top recommendations.

Minneapolis-St. Paul International Airport

1. Burger King (Concourses E, F, M)

See p. 289 for top recommendations.

2. 360 Gourmet Burrito (Concourse M)

PICK	CALORIES
Cajun Prawns Salad	290
Mediterranean Prawns Salad	290
Classic 360 Smoked Tofu Salad	319
Teriyaki Steak Salad	323
Teriyaki Chicken Breast Salad	346

SKIP	CALORIES
Cajun Steak Quesadilla	914
Thai Chicken Wrap	904
Cajun Steak Wrap	855
360 Gourmet Burrito (original)	610

3. Chili's Too (Concourses G, M)

See pp. 289–90 for top recommendations.

4. Subway (Concourse G)

See pp. 294–295 for top recommendations.

5. Starbucks (Concourses C, G, M, Baggage Claim)

See p. 294 for top recommendations.

6. Maui Tacos (Concourse C)

See p. 291 for top recommendations

7. McDonald's (Concourse G)

See p. 292 for top recommendations.

8. California Pizza Kitchen

See p. 289 for top recommendations.

John F. Kennedy International Airport (JFK)/New York

1. McDonald's (Food Court, Terminals 1, 4, 7)

See p. 292 for top recommendations.

2. Starbucks (Terminals 2, 3)

See p. 294 for top recommendations.

3. Balducci's (Terminal 2)

(calories not provided by company)

BREAKFAST

PICK

Assorted yogurts (Dannon)

Fruit salad

SKIP

Assorted baked goods

LUNCH

PICK

Chicken Caesar salad (request no croutons, and balsamic vinaigrette on the side)

Tri Color Salad (request balsamic vinaigrette on the side)

Tomato mozzarella salad

Grab and Go Fruit and Vegetable Snacks: celery and carrot sticks

Fruit: bananas, apples, oranges

Energy bars: Gnu banana walnut, cinnamon raisin fiber, or orange cranberry fiber

---
SKIP

Turkey and cheddar sandwich

Moroccan couscous

Caprese Ficelle

4. French Meadow Bakery and Café (Terminal 2)

(calories not provided by company)

PICK

Vegan Black Bean Chili

Spa Salad

Steamed mussels

Zone Organic Omelet (made with egg whites)

Tofu Scrambler Plate

Seasonal fresh fruit

Roasted vegetable sandwich on "Atkins and Zone Friendly" bread*

Free-range turkey burger on "Atkins and Zone Friendly" bread*

Veggie burger on "Atkins and Zone Friendly" bread*

SKIP

Tuna melt

BLT wrap

5. Burger King (Terminal 3)

See p. 289 for top recommendations.

6. Chili's Too / To Go (Terminal 3)

See pp. 289–90 for top recommendations.

7. Manchu Wok (Terminal 3)

See p. 291 for top recommendations.

8. Au Bon Pain (Terminals 4, 8, 9)

See pp. 288–89 for top recommendations.

9. Boar's Head Deli/Sandwiches (Terminal 6, 8)

PICK

Fresh soups, salads, and sandwiches made to order *(Use deli guidelines, pp. 225–26.)*

10. Create Your Own Salad (Terminal 6)

Stick to salad bar guidelines, p. 233.

11. Subway (Terminal 7)

See pp. 294–295 for top recommendations.

Other Basic Deli Options Located within JFK

7th Avenue Deli (Terminal 7)
Brooklyn National Deli (Terminal 9)

*Order a side of mixed greens instead of chips with sandwiches.

LaGuardia Airport/New York

1. Au Bon Pain (US Airways Terminal/Central Terminal Building)
See pp. 288–89 for top recommendations.

2. McDonald's (US Airways Terminal)
See p. 292 for top recommendations.

3. Così Pronto (Central Terminal Building)
See p. 290 for top recommendations.

4. Wendy's (Central Terminal Building)
See p. 295 for top recommendations.

Newark Liberty International Airport

1. Burger King (Terminal A)
See p. 289 for top recommendations.

2. McDonald's (Terminal B)
See p. 292 for top recommendations.

3. Au Bon Pain (Terminal C)
See pp. 288–89 for top recommendations.

4. Starbucks (Terminals A, B, C)
See p. 294 for top recommendations.

5. A & W All American Food (Terminal C)

PICK	CALORIES
Plain hot dog	180
Chili bowl	190
Grilled chicken sandwich	340

SKIP	CALORIES
Original bacon double cheeseburger	800
Chicken strips (3 pieces) with ranch dip	660

6. Maui Tacos (Terminal C)
See p. 291 for top recommendations.

7. Steak Escape (Terminal C)

PICK	CALORIES
Side salad with grilled chicken	177
With balsamic vinaigrette (90)	267
Sandwich (7"), portobello vegetarian	311
Sandwich (7"), turkey Philly	365

SKIP	CALORIES
Loaded Smashed Potatoes, bacon and cheddar	636
Sandwich (12"), meatball sub	1118

San Francisco International Airport

1. Burger King (Terminal 3)
See p. 289 for top recommendations.

2. Ebisu (International Terminal G Food Court)
(calories not provided by company)

PICK
Miso soup
Edamame
Ohitashi
Seaweed salad
Salmon teriyaki
Rolls such as Ebisu Maki (salmon with vegetables) or Kappa (cucumber)
Sashimi (such as tuna, yellowtail, salmon)

SKIP
Seafood tempura
Prawn tempura
Fried oysters

3. Firewood Café/Grill (International Terminal Boarding Area A)
(calories not provided by company)

PICK
Garden Salad with 3 fixings (salads are made to order and include basic veggies; consumers can choose 3 additional ingredients) (*recommended fixings*: broccoli, green apples, roasted chicken, button mushrooms, roasted beets) (*recommended salad dressings*: Firewood herb vinaigrette, low-fat creamy garlic)

Mixed green salad

Herb roasted chicken (½ order) (ask for mixed green salad instead of potatoes)

SKIP

Penne in White Wine Cream Sauce

Baked Rigatoni

Garden salad fixings to skip: candied walnuts, blue cheese

Garden salad dressings to skip: classic Caesar

4. Mission Bar & Grill

(calories not provided by company)

PICK

Fruit Bowl

Vegetarian Scramble (order without home fries, with wheat toast, and use jam on toast)

House salad (add grilled chicken and order with balsamic dressing)

Veggie burger (order side salad instead of fries, use mustard or ketchup instead of mayo)

Grilled chicken breast sandwich served on wheat bun (skip fries, use mustard or ketchup instead of mayo)

SKIP

Quesadilla with Steak

Club Sandwich and Fries

Cheesesteak Sandwich and Fries

Chicken Strips and Fries

5. San Francisco Soup Company (Terminal 3)

PICK	CALORIES
Tomato basil	140
Minestrone	141
Grandma Mary's Chicken Soup	159
Creole vegetable	165
Grilled chicken artichoke	169
Mixed greens salad	324

SKIP	CALORIES
Grilled chicken Caesar salad	651
New England clam chowder	486
Hummus wrap (½ sandwich)	460
Broccoli cheddar soup	404

6. Subway (Terminal 3 Boarding Area E)
See pp. 294–95 for top recommendations.

7. Yankee Pier (Terminal 3)
(calories not provided by company)
This is a sample menu only. Menu changes seasonally.

PICK

Mixed green salad with lemon-basil vinaigrette

Jumbo prawns (raw bar)

Bradley's Caesar Salad (order without croutons and with vinaigrette instead)

Yankee Salad with grilled salmon, Fuji apple, blue cheese (order without blue cheese and with vinaigrette)

Today's catch (grilled fish option) with 2 sides (recommend selecting steamed vegetables and sautéed spinach)

Grilled free-range chicken breast served with whipped potatoes, spinach (order without potatoes)

SKIP

Popcorn shrimp

Fish and Chips

Crab cake sandwich and fries

Sourdough French toast with orange caramel syrup

Hong Kong International Airport

1. Oliver's Super Sandwiches (SkyMart, Terminal 1)
(Calories not provided by company)

PICK

"Create Your Own Sandwich" (choose whole wheat sliced bread, smoked turkey or roasted chicken, and American mustard)

Herb roasted chicken Caesar salad (ask for dressing on the side)

Italian Vegetable Soup (8 oz)

Fresh fruit salad

Roast beef and cheddar on a whole wheat baguette

Daily Delicious Pasta

2. The Spaghetti House (SkyMart, Terminal 1)
(calories not provided by company)

PICK

Caesar salad with shrimp*

Caesar salad with herb grilled chicken breast*

Grilled herb chicken breast with mixed vegetables salad*

Minestrone soup

SKIP

Fettuccine with Cream Seafood Deluxe

Italian Special Pizza

3. Popeyes Chicken & Biscuits (SkyMart, Terminal 1)
See p. 293 for top recommendations.

4. Pret A Manger (SkyPlaza, Terminal 2)

SKIP	CALORIES
Vegetable goulash	103
Minestrone soup	152
Ratatouille	160
Mango Fruit Fool	171
Avocado formaggio sandwich	197
Tuna Niçoise salad	232
Coronation Chicken Sandwich	248
Ham, cheese, and pickle sandwich	266
Crayfish and roquette wrap	271

SKIP	CALORIES
Avocado Pinenut Wrap	484
Brie, tomato, and basil Brioche	492

5. Burger King (SkyMart, Terminal 1; Sky Plaza, Terminal 2)
See p. 289 for top recommendations.

6. A Hereford Beefstouw
(calories not provided by company)

* For salads ask for Italian dressing on the side.

Shrimp cocktail

Caesar salad (ask for dressing on the side)

Grilled king prawns (200 g)

Australian filet steak (140 g) (no sides or butter)

SKIP

Rack of lamb

Pan-fried goose liver served with mango salad

London Heathrow Airport

1. Caffe Nero (Terminals 1, 2, 3, 4)

PICK	CALORIES
Classic Fruit Salad	75
Tuna Niçoise salad	236
Chicken with oven-roasted tomatoes and spinach (on low-fat malted wheat grain bread)	320
Prawns with lemon dressing and rocket salad (on wholemeal bread)	342
SKIP	
Italian meatballs with tomato sauce panini	449
Italian tuna melt panini	463

2. Pret A Manger (Terminals 1, 2, 3, 4)

PICK	CALORIES
Miso soup	46
Slim Pret, Wild Crayfish and Rocket Sandwich	185
Slim Pret, Chicken "Hail" Caesar	214
Slim Pret, Chicken Avocado Sandwich	228
Salmon Nigiri	245
Vegetarian sushi	269
Slim Pret, Classic Superclub Sandwich	274
Herb Chicken Salad Wrap	315

SKIP	CALORIES
New York Cheddar Club Sandwich	641
Swedish Meatball Ragu Hot Wrap	566

3. Est Est Est (Terminals 1, 2, 3, 4)
(calories not provided by company)

PICK

Steamed mussels with white wine, garlic, and parsley

Caesar salad with chicken (ask for dressing on the side, use 2 T)

EST house mixed salad

Chargrilled chicken breast with lemon and garlic (order a side of steamed broccoli)

Steamed sea bass with roasted sweet potato, chili, lemon, and thyme

SKIP

Penne pasta in a creamy carbonara sauce

Veal cutlet with cured ham and sage served with baked rosemary potatoes

Any of the pizzas

4. Costa (Terminals 1, 2, 3, 4)

PICK	CALORIES
Italian ham salad sandwich	277
<5% Fat Roast Chicken Sandwich	306
<5% Fat Tuna Salad Sandwich	310
Low-fat Malted Arrabiata Chicken Sandwich	363

SKIP	CALORIES
Bacon Massimo Panini	590
Tuna Melt Panini	544

5. Eat (Terminal 3)

PICK	CALORIES
Gazpacho	78
Old-fashioned Chicken and Egg Noodle Soup	116
French onion soup	156
Moroccan Chicken and Root Vegetable Soup	220
Vegetarian sushi	240
Fish sushi	308
EAT Superfood Salad	334
Tuna and red onion sandwich	361

SKIP	CALORIES
Thai Chicken Sandwich	669
EAT Club	873

6. Ponti's (Terminal 3)

(calories not provided by company)

PICK
Ponti's Minestrone Soup
"Create Your Own" Sandwich (choose brown bread and either chargrilled chicken breast, or tuna)
Crayfish and rocket salad (ask for no croutons and dressing on the side)
Chicken Caesar salad (ask for no croutons and dressing on the side)

SKIP
Lasagna al Forno
Pizza Pepperoni

7. Starbucks (Terminals 3, 4)

See p. 294 for top recommendations.

Recommendations at Common Airport Chains

Au Bon Pain

BREAKFAST

PICK	CALORIES
Arugula and tomato frittata	290
Ham and cheddar frittata	320

SKIP	CALORIES
Chocolate chunk muffin	590
Plain bagel with egg, cheese, and bacon	560
Breakfast Prosciutto Sandwich	660

LUNCH

PICK	CALORIES
Southwest Vegetable Soup (medium)	100
Thai Chicken Salad	190
With fat-free raspberry vinaigrette (80)	270
Caesar salad	210
With fat-free raspberry vinaigrette (80)	290

Burger King

PICK	CALORIES
Side garden salad	15
With Ken's fat-free ranch dressing (60)	75
Croissan'wich Egg & Cheese (without the croissant)	150
Hamburger (without the bun)	160
Hamburger	290
TenderGrill Chicken Garden Salad (without dressing)	240
With Ken's fat-free ranch dressing (60)	300

KIDS' MENU PICK	CALORIES
Flame-broiled Chicken Tenders (4-piece serving)	145
BK Fresh Apple Fries	35
BK Kids Meal (Chicken Tenders, Apple Fries, and low-fat milk)	305

SKIP	CALORIES
Chocolate milk shake, king	1260
Triple Whopper sandwich	1130
BK Quad Stacker	1000

California Pizza Kitchen

PICK

Chinese chicken salad (skip the crispy wontons and use only 1 spoonful of the dressing)

Chicken Caesar (skip the croutons and use only 1 spoonful of the dressing)

Chili's

PICK (FROM GUILTLESS GRILL)	CALORIES
Side steamed veggies with Parmesan cheese	60
Black bean burger patty only (no bun or topping)	200
With whole wheat bun (90)	290
Guiltless Salmon	480
Guiltless Chicken Sandwich	490

Grilled chicken Caesar salad (without croutons and balsamic vinaigrette instead of Caesar dressing, calories not available)

SKIP	CALORIES
Smoked Turkey sandwich	930
Bacon burger	1080
Chicken Ranch Sandwich	1150
Awesome Blossom with Seasoned Sauce	2710

Così

BREAKFAST

PICK	CALORIES
Fruit salad	216

SKIP	CALORIES
Granola cereal	564
Apple crumb cake	540

LUNCH

PICK	CALORIES
Caesar salad	182
Pollo E Pasta Soup Bowl	183
Shanghai Chicken Salad	221
With fat-free balsamic vinaigrette	227
With low-fat ginger soy dressing	295
Brie and fruit plate	277

SKIP	CALORIES
Roasted turkey and brie sandwich	772
Tuna cheddar melt	956

Manchu Wok

All five-ounce servings.

PICK	CALORIES
Garlic Green Beans	117
Mixed vegetables	130
Satay Chicken	211
Oriental Grilled Chicken	255
Green Bean Chicken	258
Beef and Broccoli	271
Orange Chicken	279
Honey Garlic Chicken	326

SKIP	CALORIES
Sweet and Sour Chicken	450
BBQ Pork	427
Sesame Chicken	415

Maui Tacos

PICK	CALORIES
Rock Shrimp Salad	170
Chopped Tuna Salad	275
Vegetarian Bowl	390

SKIP	CALORIES
Napili Burrito	755
Chicken Mango Salad	605
Chicken Combo Platter with black beans	610

Max & Erma's

Max & Erma's provides nutrition information only for "No Guilt" menu offerings.

PICK (BEST "NO GUILT" CHOICES)	CALORIES
Fruit salad	54
Baby Greens Salad (without breadstick)	119
With low-fat Tex Mex dressing (23)	142
With fat-free honey mustard (60)	179
Shrimp Stack Salad	322
Half Hula Bowl (with fat-free honey mustard dressing)	366

SKIP	CALORIES
Black Bean Roll-Ups	577
Full Hula Bowl (without breadstick)	576

McDonald's

BREAKFAST

PICK	CALORIES
McDonald's Fruit 'n Yogurt Parfait (without granola)	130
Egg McMuffin (without the English Muffin)	160

SKIP	CALORIES
Deluxe Breakfast	1320
Hotcakes and sausage	780

LUNCH/DINNER

PICK	CALORIES
Side salad	20
With low-fat balsamic vinaigrette (40)	60
McDonald's Hamburger (without the bun)	90
Fruit and walnut salad (snack size)	210
With low-fat balsamic vinaigrette (40)	250
McDonald's Hamburger	250
Caesar salad with grilled chicken	220
With low-fat balsamic vinaigrette (40)	260
Honey Mustard Snack Wrap (grilled chicken)	260
Asian Salad with Grilled Chicken	300
With low-fat balsamic vinaigrette (40)	340

SKIP	CALORIES
Double Quarter Pounder with Cheese	740
With medium French fries (380)	1120
Premium Crispy Chicken Club Sandwich	660

Panda Express

PICK	CALORIES
Mixed Veggies	70
Veggie Spring Roll (1 piece)	80
Hot and Sour Soup	110
Mushroom Chicken	130
Broccoli Beef	150
Tangy Shrimp	150
Chicken Breast with String Beans	160
Eggplant and Tofu in Garlic Sauce	180
Black Pepper Chicken	200
Kung Pao Shrimp	240
Mandarin Chicken	250

SKIP	CALORIES
Orange Chicken	500
BBQ Pork	440

Note: All chicken, beef, and shrimp dishes listed are served as 5.5-oz portions. Skip rice.

Popeyes Chicken & Biscuits

PICK THE BREAST PLUS EITHER THE THIGH, WING, OR LEG AND A SIDE OF GREEN BEANS	CALORIES
Mild or spicy chicken breast (skinless and breading removed)	120
Mild or spicy chicken thigh (skinless and breading removed)	80
Mild or spicy chicken wing (skinless and breading removed)	40
Mild or spicy chicken leg (skinless and breading removed)	50
Green beans side	70

SKIP	CALORIES
Deluxe Sandwich with mayo	630
Chicken and Sausage Jambalaya	660

Starbucks

Available in participating stores, offerings vary regionally.

PICK	CALORIES
Any version of non- or low-fat yogurt	60–160
Any breakfast wrap or sandwich under 300 calories	200–300
Reduced fat turkey bacon, egg, and reduced fat white cheddar sandwich	350

SKIP	CALORIES
Classic Sausage, Egg & Cheddar	470
Scones (various flavors)	480–500
Regular muffins (not low/reduced fat)	420–500

LUNCH

Available in participating stores, offerings vary regionally.

PICK	CALORIES
Low-fat turkey and artichoke sandwich	190
Tomato Mozzarella Insalata	280
Turkey and Swiss sandwich (no condiments)	280
Asian-style layered salad	310
Vegetable vinaigrette	310
Very Veggie Crunch Wrap	310
Fiesta Salad	320
Fruit and cheese plate	370

SKIP	CALORIES
Chicken cheddar club with bacon	550
Egg salad on multigrain	470
Garden tuna salad wrap	460

Subway

PICK	CALORIES
Jared (low-fat) Salads: ham, roast beef, club, turkey breast, or Veggie Delite	150 (or less)
Any above salad with fat-free Italian Dressing (35)	185 (or less)

6" Jared (low-fat) Sandwiches:

PICK	CALORIES
Veggie Delite	230
Turkey breast	280
Ham	290
Roast beef	290
Oven-roasted chicken breast	310

Note: These do not include dressings or sauces. Suggest mustard or vinegar to keep calories low.

SKIP	CALORIES
6" Double Meatball Marinara Sub	860
6" Double Subway Steak and Cheese Sub	540

Wendy's

PICK	CALORIES
Wendy's Mandarin Chicken Salad (without noodles or almonds)	170
With fat-free French dressing (70)	240
Small chili	220
Wendy's Jr. Hamburger	280
Wendy's Grilled Chicken Sandwich	310

SKIP	
Southwest Taco Salad with Ancho Chipotle Ranch Dressing	680
Wendy's Old Fashioned Burgers: ½ lb Double with Cheese	700

Airline Meals

Getting nutritional information from the airlines about their meals is an exercise in frustration. Most are far from forthcoming about what they're serving you in the air. Some don't seem to have any nutritional information at all; others don't want to share it. We did the best we could and have been able to come up with some good general recommendations on what to choose on your flight. Keep in mind that the airlines offer varying meals regionally and that they change them regularly so that an entrée offered in May might be off the menu in August. And a meal on a flight from Denver may not be offered on a flight from Boston.

Some general guidelines for flying Wall Streeters: for most airlines, you can call ahead and pick a low-calorie, low-fat, or low-cholesterol meal, if a meal is served. You can also call or check the airline website to find out if a meal will be served, or just snacks. In first class and business class, meals are typically served, but you need to steer clear of Dry Carbs, salty nuts, salty drinks. If you eat just the protein, veggies, and fruit, the meal itself can be nutritious. You may want to bring along snacks on your trip. You should make your choices based on what kind of eater you are: a Controlled Eater or a

Clean Plate Clubber. See the travel chapter, page 144, for more details on this.

Airlines are all domestic and are in alphabetical order.

American Airlines

American sells snacks and meals. On flights over three hours your breakfast option is a breakfast bagel sandwich. You can take out the turkey and cheese and have it with Dijonnaise mustard and eat half the bagel (about 330 calories), but you have to be a good deconstructor and a Controlled Eater. If you ate the bagel breakfast sandwich as it is served with the mustard, it would be about 470 calories. On flights over three hours in the afternoon or evening there is also an Asian chicken salad served without the dressing for around 360 calories. There are individual snacks offered, but all are between 300 and 860 calories, so best to skip.

Note: These calorie counts are just estimates, as portion sizes are not available for the meals.

INDIVIDUAL SNACKS AVAILABLE ON AMERICAN AIRLINES ($3 EACH)

- Great Nut Supply (4 oz) (650–700 calories, 170 calories/oz)
- Mega Bite Cookie (4 oz) (250–300 calories)
- Lay's Stax Potato Crisps (5.75 oz) (860 calories, 150 calories/oz)
- M&M's (5.3 oz) (730 calories, 138 calories/oz)
- 3 Musketeers (300 calories)

EXAMPLES OF FRESH LIGHT MEALS AVAILABLE FOR $5

- Breakfast Bagel Sandwich (plain bagel [260], slices of roasted turkey breast [80], mild Muenster cheese [100], side of mayonnaise [150], Dijonnaise mustard [25]) (estimated 600 calories with mayo, estimated 470 calories with mustard)
- Asian Chicken Salad (Romaine lettuce [16], napa cabbage [13], grilled chicken [120], water chestnuts [60], red peppers [20], mandarin oranges [40], slivered almonds [100], oriental sesame dressing on side [140]) (estimated 500 calories with dressing, estimated 360 calories without dressing)

American Airlines also offers the following special meals available by preorder:

- **Diabetic**
- **Gluten-free**
- **Vegetarian**

Continental Airlines

Continental is the only airline that serves meals at meal times on flights longer than two hours. Meal includes a sandwich—smoked turkey, oven roasted turkey, roast beef, or ham and cheese—on freshly baked white or wheat rolls, and a sweet item (Almond Delight, Smores Russell Stover, Pecan Delight), with either carrot sticks or chips. The sandwiches are all pretty plain and add up to about 200 calories. Skip the chocolate bar, peanuts, and pretzels, and enjoy the carrots.

COLD SANDWICH
- **Turkey sandwich (2 slices Jennie'O Smoked Turkey Breast [1.4 oz, 40 calories], small greenleaf lettuce leaf [5], 1.5-oz French petit pain roll [90], 1 packet of Hellmann's Light Mayo [35]) (170 calories total)**
- **Ham sandwich (1 slice of smoked ham [1 oz, 103 calories], small greenleaf lettuce leaf [5], 1.5-oz French petit pain roll [90], 1 packet of French's Yellow Mustard [3]) (201 calories total)**
- **1 small bag of carrots (35 calories)**

DESSERT
- **1 Twix Cookie Fun Size Candy Bar (80 calories)**

OTHER SNACKS (SHORTER FLIGHTS)
- **1.5-oz bag of honey-roasted peanuts (80 calories)**
  or
- **1.5-oz bag of mini pretzels (50 calories)**

Continental also offers special meals that may be preordered, including:

- **Vegan**
- **Diabetic**

- **Gluten-free**
- **Low-calorie**
- **Low-fat/low-cholesterol**
- **Low-sodium**

Delta Air Lines

On flights between 1.5 and 3.5 hours you'll find a Snack Basket. Your best bet is a Quaker granola bar. On longer flights, over 3.5 hours, there is a snack that is suitable only for Controlled Eaters (I speak from experience here: I ate it all!). Pick the cheese spread and cranberry/golden raisin mix (skip the crackers and cookie).

CLASS OF SERVICE	LESS THAN 450 MILES (LESS THAN 1.5 HOURS)	BETWEEN 450 AND 1550 MILES (1.5–3.5 HOURS)	1550 MILES OR MORE (3.5 HOURS OR MORE)
Economy Class	1 snack item available (items may vary)	Choice of 1 item from Snack Basket	Snack and choice of 1 item from Snack Basket
First Class	Choice of items from Snack Basket	Choice of items from Snack Basket	Choice of items from Snack Basket and complimentary meal service

SNACK CHOICES

Certain flights offer "Choice of items from Snack Basket," which includes:

- **Frito-Lay Sun Chips (140 calories)**
- **Quaker Granola Bars (120 calories)**
- **Dry-roasted peanuts (170 calories)**
- **Biscoff Cookies (146 calories)**
- **Lance Honey Peanut Butter Crackers (190 calories)**

On longer flights, a "Snack" is served, which includes:

- **Parmesan Peppercorn Cheese Spread (70 calories)**
- **Pepperidge Farm Crackers (100 calories)**
- **Cranberry/golden raisin mix (90 calories)**
- **Walker's Chocolate Chip Shortbread Cookie (150 calories)**

Meal Choices

Delta also offers the following special meals for order on flights where complimentary meal service is offered:

- **Bland**
- **Diabetic**
- **Kosher**
- **Low-sodium**
- **Vegetarian**

JetBlue

They have a few snack choices, including hundred-calorie packs of Wheat Thins. For those who are protein-starved, go for the all-nuts cashew halves, 170 calories. They give you only one snack at a time, so this may be a good choice for Controlled Eaters and Clean Plate Clubbers who love plane food and come empty-handed. But take only one!

Snack Choices

- **Nabisco 100-Calorie Packs Wheat Thins Minis (100 calories)**
- **Chocobillys Chocolate Chunk (130 calories)**
- **Doritos Munchies Mix (140 calories)**
- **Mama Says Biscotti Gingerbread Grande (210 calories)**
- **Mama Says Biscotti Pistachio Grande (150 calories)**
- **Mrs. Good Cookie Jungle Crackers (120 calories)**
- **Terra Blues Potato Chips (140 calories)**
- **All Nuts Jumbo Cashew Halves (170 calories)**

United Airlines

On flights over three hours, United has snack choice boxes that have some healthy options, but they range from 560 to 895 calories (the highest-calorie one being trans-fat-free and vegetarian) if you eat everything in the box. If you end up with a box in front of you, I would pick two choices and make it a protein and look for a fruit (cheese and apple-sauce, or tuna and raisins, or double up on the protein with cheese and beef jerky). They also have a wrap/sandwich/turkey salad option, but you need to deconstruct the sandwich—eating just the protein—or in the salad, pick out the lettuce, turkey, approved veggies, and have some fruit on the side. You basically have to be a Controlled Eater in this situation and good at navigating your way though each possibility to make the healthiest choice. If you are not a good deconstructor, the best choice would be the turkey wrap at 425 calories (call it your Juicy Carb for the day). Total calories: Smartpack, 895; Minimeal, 560; Quickpick, 735; Ritebite, 625. Cost: $5 per box.

SMARTPACK

Total calories: 895 (but trans-fat-free and vegetarian)

- **SunGold Creamy SunButter (266 calories)**
- **Bear Naked All-Natural Fruit and Nut Granola (280 calories)**
- **Vermont Village Cannery Organic Peach Applesauce (80 calories)**
- **Cowbell Cheese White Cheddar Cheese (50 calories)**
- **Pita Shack Multigrain and Honey Lavash Crackers (120 calories)**
- **Hero Strawberry Preserves (64 calories)**
- **Bali's Best Latte Candy (15 calories)**
- **Emer'gen-C Fizzing Drink Mix (20 calories)**

MINIMEAL

Total calories: 560

- **Hormel Hard Salami Slices (110 calories)**
- **Rondelé Peppercorn Parmesan Cheese Spread (70 calories)**
- **Venus Wheat Crackers (60 calories)**
- **Mott's Healthy Harvest Granny Smith Applesauce, unsweetened (50 calories)**
- **Kettle Classics Natural Potato Chips (150 calories)**
- **Pepperidge Farm Milano Cookies (120 calories)**

QUICKPICK

Total calories: 735

- **Jack Link's Hickory-smoked Beef Jerky (60 calories)**
- **Just the Cheese Baked Cheddar Cheese Snacks (75 calories)**

- Stoned Classics All-natural Blue Tortilla Chips (180 calories)

- La Victoria Thick n' Chunky Salsa (15 calories)

- SunRise Honey-coated Trail Mix (205.5 calories)

- Mrs. Fields Milk Chocolate-Chip Cookie (200 calories)

RITEBITE

Total calories: 625

- Bumblebee Sensations Lemon and Pepper Seasoned Tuna Medley (110 calories)

- Late July Organic Crackers (100 calories)

- Wild Garden Hummus (73.5 calories)

- Stacy's Multigrain Baked Pita Chips (130 calories)

- Fino Selections Gouda Cheese (101 calories)

- Newman's Own Organic California Raisins (45.5 calories)

- Mini-Toblerone (66.5 calories)

Meals

Sample meals (available for purchase) are posted on United's website. Here are estimated calories for a few of them:

- *Trader Vic's Turkey Wrap* (sliced mesquite turkey breast [80], iceberg lettuce [15], sliced cucumber [8], wasabi mayonnaise [150 for 1.5 T], fresh tortilla wrap [170]) (425 calories total)

- *Maui Chicken Sandwich* (grilled sliced chicken breast [175], topped with provolone cheese [100], sliced red onion [15], crisp iceberg lettuce [15], chutney mayonnaise blend [150], served on Asiago cheese roll [225]) (680 calories total)

- *Harvest Moon Chopped Turkey Salad* (Romaine lettuce [25], roasted turkey breast [150], chopped walnuts [150], apples [50], tomatoes [35], crumbled blue cheese [110], bacon [100], dried cranberries [120], olives [35], Asian sesame ginger dressing [140], with selection of fresh seasonal fruit [60]) (975 calories total)

United also offers the following special medical diets that need to be preordered:

- Diabetic
- Low-purine
- Low-fat/low-cholesterol

- **Low-calorie**
- **High-fiber**
- **Low-protein**
- **Low-sodium**
- **Gluten-free**

Wall Street Shopping List

P lease note that the foods marked with a "Maintenance Only" are for people on Maintenance; "CE" refers to Controlled Eaters; CPC refers to Clean Plate Club Eaters.

The Template List

1. Juicy Carbs

JUICY VEGGIE CARBS (SIZE OF FIST)

- **Baked white or sweet potato (sweet is healthier option and best CPC choice)**
- **Beans (black/kidney)**
- **Lentils**
- **Chickpeas (no hummus allowed)**
- **Corn**
- **Winter squash**
- **Peas**

BREAD

For CE only.

- Sahara Whole Wheat Pita
- Thomas' Light Multi-Grain English Muffin
- Weight Watchers 100% Whole Wheat Pita (2 oz)
- Arnold's Bakery Light

WAFFLES

- Kashi Go Lean Waffles (2/serving, Maintenance Only)
- Van's Organic Original Waffles (2/serving, Maintenance Only)

OTHER GRAINS

- Unprocessed bran (Quaker or Hodgson Mill)
- Quinoa, couscous, barley, brown rice
- Flaxseeds (ground)

2. Fiber

COLD CEREAL

Must follow servings on box (and CPC can only have mixed into yogurt).

- Uncle Sam Original
- Arrowhead Mills Shredded Wheat, bite-sized
- Nutritious Living Hi-Lo
- Nature's Path Flax Plus
- Nutritious Living Dr. Sears Zone Cereal, honey almond
- Kashi Go Lean Original
- Nature's Path Optimum Slim
- Kashi Organic Promise Autumn Wheat
- Back to Nature Banana Nut Multibran
- Kashi Good Friends
- General Mill's Fiber One Original
- Kellogg's All-Bran Original or All-Bran Bran Buds

OATMEAL/HOT CEREAL

- Quaker Instant Oatmeal, regular
- Quaker Instant Oatmeal, weight control packets (CPC)
- Quaker low-sugar flavored oatmeal packets (CPC)
- Arrowhead Mills Instant Oatmeal

- McCann's Irish Oatmeal
- McCann's Instant Sugar-Free Irish Oatmeal (Comes in boxes of 8 packs, in cinnamon roll, maple and brown sugar flavor, and apples and cinnamon)
- Kashi Go Lean Hot Cereal (CPC)

CRACKERS

- Fiber Rich crackers *(www.fiberrich.bigstep.com)* (CPC)
- GG Scandinavian Bran Crispbread (CPC)
- Wasa Fiber Rye Crispbread
- Wasa Crisp'n Light 7-Grain Crackerbreads

HIGH-FIBER WRAPS FOR CPC OR CE

- La Tortilla Factory (regular or large original flavor) *(www.latortillafactory.com/jadworks/ltf/jwsuite.nsf/sitewelcome/Home)*

ADDITIONAL HIGH-FIBER WRAP OPTIONS FOR CE ONLY

- Mission Carb Balance Whole Wheat, fajita size
- Damascus (whole wheat or flax) roll-ups
- Tumaro's Low-in-Carbs Tortilla
- Trader Joe's Low-carb Wrap
- Aladdin Low-carb Wrap

3. Fruits

- Fresh fruit, your choice. Choose any of the following (check servings on the plan): apple, apricots, blueberries, raspberries, strawberries, cantaloupe, grapefruit, clementines, honeydew, orange, peach, plum, nectarine, pineapple, small banana, cherries (CE only), grapes (CE only).
- Frozen fruit: any brand without sauce or added ingredients. One good choice is Cascadian Farms organic frozen berries.

4. Vegetables

FRESH

- Fresh veggies, your choice. Choose any of the following: asparagus, artichoke hearts, broccoli, beets (CE only), cabbage, cauliflower, celery, chard, collard greens, cucumbers, escarole, eggplant, fennel, green beans, green onions, kale, lettuce, mushrooms, peppers, spinach, sprouts, tomato (CE only), zucchini, carrots (CE only), eggplant.

- Earthbound Farm organic produce is recommended. (Greens are triple-washed, making salad prep easier.)
- Large Romaine lettuce leaves (good for sandwich option instead of wrap)

FROZEN

- Cascadian Farms organic frozen vegetables
- Birds Eye Steamfresh
- Green Giant Simply Steam no sauce
- Any brand frozen spinach, broccoli, or cauliflower (prepare in Ziploc Zip 'n Steam cooking bags)

5. Protein

MEAT/FISH OPTIONS

Clients often ask me if the breaded (Bell & Evans and Perdue) chicken breasts are a carb. They are only lightly breaded and so I don't count them as carbs. But you must keep to only one serving, as listed on the package, if you choose them.

- Murray's organic boneless skinless chicken breast
- Bell & Evans air-chilled breaded chicken breast (uncooked)
- Perdue low-fat breaded chicken cutlet (fully cooked)
- 4 1/4-lb bags of fresh turkey breast (Applegate Farms or any other low-sodium version at the deli counter) (a must for CPC)
- Honeysuckle White 99% fat-free ground turkey
- Jennie-O Turkey Store lean turkey burgers
- Any seafood (salmon, sole, tilapia, halibut, orange ruffy, shrimp, scallops)
- Starkist tuna in water in a pouch (canned in water works as well)
- Bilinski's Gourmet Low-fat Chicken Sausage
- Applegate Farms chicken and apple sausage
- Casual Gourmet chicken sausages
- Buffalo Burger

EGG OPTIONS

- Eggology on-the-Go 100% Egg Whites (4 oz, microwavable)
- Better'n Eggs ReddiEgg
- All Whites (by Papetti Foods)
- Egg Beaters
- Eggs of your choice (good to hard boil in advance or for making omelets at home)

DAIRY OPTIONS

YOGURT

- Fage Greek Yogurt, 0% fat (5.7 oz) or 2% fat (7 oz)
- Dannon Light & Fit (smoothies included)
- Stonyfield Farm Organic Light Smoothies
- Stonyfield Farm Non-fat Fruit-Flavored Yogurt
- Stonyfield Farm Oikos Organic 0% Fat Greek Yogurt

CHEESE

FOR CPC ONLY IF CHEESE IS NOT A TRIGGER.

- Laughing Cow Light cheese (Mini Babybel Light, or any of the "Light" variety wedges)
- Polly-O String Cheese, part skim or 2%
- Horizon or Kraft part skim or reduced fat shredded cheese
- Kraft 2% or fat-free cheese slices
- Galaxy Nutritional Foods Veggie Slices
- Organic Valley Stringles, mozzarella (part skim)
- Cabot's ¾-oz reduced fat mini cheddar bars

COTTAGE CHEESE

- Breakstones (2% snack size) (CPC)
- Friendship 1%
- Friendship whipped 1%
- Light & Lively (0% snack size) (CPC)

MILK

- Skim
- Skim plus
- Silk Unsweetened Soymilk
- 8th Continent Fat-Free Soymilk, original
- Organic Valley Family of Farms 1% low-fat milk (unrefrigerated, in 8-oz box, good for office or travel)

6. Beverages

- Smartwater

- Low-sodium V8 juice or tomato juice

- True Lemon *(http://www.truelemon.com/)*

- Green tea

- Flavored/plain seltzer (sodium-free)

- Herbal tea, your choice

- Swiss Miss Sugar-Free Hot Cocoa Mix

- Ghirardelli Chocolate Premium Hot Cocoa

7. Condiments

SEASONINGS

Many of my clients love to grill in the summer and ask for recommendations on grills and marinades, and that's why I include the Williams-Sonoma Grilling Rub. The taco mix is good for making low-fat turkey tacos. If you use the extra-lean ground turkey, prepare with mix, and serve with shredded lettuce, tomato, onion on a La Tortilla wrap, you've got a delicious, low-fat taco.

- All fresh herbs and dry spices

- Mrs. Dash

- Cinnamon

- Vanilla extract

- Splenda

- Williams-Sonoma Grilling Rub (poultry or fish)

- Old El Paso Taco Mix (40% less sodium)

SALAD DRESSINGS
- Annie's Naturals low-fat ginger

- Newman's Own light balsamic

- Newman's Own light Italian

- Maple Grove Farms fat-free balsamic vinaigrette

- Wish-Bone Just 2 Good Lite Italian

- Wish-Bone salad spritzers

- Balsamic vinegar

- Extra virgin olive oil
- Make your own (balsamic vinegar plus Grey Poupon made with white-wine Dijon mustard)

PEANUT BUTTER/ALMOND BUTTER
- Justin's nut butter (*justinsnutbutter.com*) (in the individual packets, CPC)
- Better 'n Peanut Butter (CE only)
- Arrowhead Mills organic (CE only)
- Any all-natural or organic brand (CE only)

SPREADS
- Benecol light
- Brummel and Brown yogurt-based butter spread
- Mustard, your choice
- Hellmann's light mayo
- Desert Pepper Trading Company spicy black bean dips (all salsas as well) (CE only)
- Smucker's sugar-free preserves (CE only)

SOUP MIX
- Knorr vegetable or onion recipe mix

COOKING/BBQ/PASTA
ALL COUNT AS JUICY CARB.
- Trader Joe's Roasted Pepita Simmer Sauce (add to stir-fried beef, chicken, or shrimp)
- Dinosaur Bar-B-Que Mojito Marinade and Dressing (marinate chicken, beef, or pork)
- KC Masterpiece Low-calorie Classic Blend BBQ Sauce
- Hafa-Dai BBQ Sauce and Marinade
- Classico Fire Roasted Tomato and Garlic Sauce
- Muir Glen Marinara Sauce

SYRUP
CE ONLY.
- Cary's Sugar-Free Syrup
- Aunt Jemima's Light

8. Fun Snacks

- **Pria bar**
  - 110 Plus
  - Complete Nutrition
  - Grain Essentials
- **Lärabar (apple pie or cherry pie)**
- **Luna bar**
- **Luna Sunrise bar**
- **Gnu bar**
- **Kashi TLC chewy granola bar**
- **Kashi Go Lean Crunchy! bar**
- **Kashi Go Lean Roll! bar**
- **Think Green bar (chocolate chip is best)**
- **EAS Myoplex Lite bar**
- **Nature Valley granola bar**
- **Balance Original bar**
- **Balance Bar**
- **ZonePerfect All-Natural Nutrition Bar (210 calories, but still OK)**
- **ZonePerfect All-Natural Nutrition Snack Size Bar**

OTHER TYPES OF FUN SNACKS

- **Glenny's**
  - 1.3-oz bag Soy Crisps
  - 100-Calorie Brownie
  - Zen Health Tortilla Crisps or Spud Delites
  - Light N' Crispy Bars
- **Quaker Crispy Delights (Chocolate Drizzle or Cinnamon Streusel)**
- **Healthy Delites Crispy Delites, 1-oz bag**
- **Orville Redenbacher's Mini Bags, 94% fat-free**
- **Jolly Time 94% fat-free mini microwave bags**
- **Boston's Lite Popcorn, precooked, individual bag**
- **VitaMuffin (2 oz tops) or VitaBrownies**
- **Laughing Cow Gourmet Cheese & Baguettes**
- **Late July organic cheddar cheese crackers/peanut butter crackers (individual bags only)**

- CocoVia chocolate bar
- Sugar-free Jell-O gelatin snacks
- Sugar-free Jell-O pudding snacks
- Shelton's Turkey Jerky (I serving packet)
- Nature Valley Fruit Crisps
- Nabisco 100-calorie packs
- All Bran Snack Bites
- Kozy Shack no-sugar-added rice pudding
- Mott's Healthy Harvest no-sugar-added applesauce cup, any flavor

LITE MORNING FUN SNACKS FOR CES
- Apple or any hand fruit
- 6 ounces Dannon Light & Fit yogurt
- 5-ounce 0% fat Greek yogurt
- I Laughing Cow Light wedge and a Fiber Rich cracker
- I Babybel Light and a Fiber Rich cracker
- 2 plain Fiber Rich crackers
- 10–12 almonds, raw, unsalted

EVENING SNACKS FOR CES
- Tofutti pops
- Edy's Fruit Bars
- Edy's No Sugar Added Fruit Bars
- Sugar Free The Original Brand Popsicle
- Fudge bar, no added sugar (various brands)
- Stonyfield Farm's squeezer—freeze the yogurt tube
- Dannon Light & Fit—freeze it

Additional Shopping List Items

Pasta Substitutes

- Kombu Seaweed Noodles
- Tofu Shirataki Noodles (sold in produce section)

Soups

Check the serving size on the soup container. If you're a CPCer, Trader Joe's or Tabatchnick's are good choices because they come in individual servings. If you're salt-sensitive, either because of high blood pressure or because you tend to bloat, then choose low-sodium soups. If the soup has beans, lentils, corn, potato, squash, peas, or barley, you must count it as a Juicy Carb. The exception is that beans/lentils count as protein if they're the only protein in meal.

- **Amy's Soups Light in Sodium Line: tomato bisque, cream of tomato, lentil veggie, minestrone**
- **Health Valley Organic "On the Go" Soups**
- **Pritikin soups**
- **Imagine broths**
- **Pacific broths**
- **Campbell's low-sodium soup**
- **Trader Joe's low-fat reduced-sodium split pea soup**
- **Trader Joe's low-fat butternut squash soup**
- **Tabatchnick soups**

Meals/Meal Components

In general, for lunch you should choose a frozen meal that's less than 280 calories for women and 300 calories for men. For dinner, choose an entrée that's less than 380 for women and less than 400 for men. If you're eating late, say after 9 P.M., it's best to choose a dinner that's very low in calories. For example, Amy's Mexican Tamale Pie is just 150 calories. This is a good late-dinner choice. I like Amy's brand because they're organic and they taste great. All frozen meals count as a Juicy Carb.

FROZEN MEALS
- **Amy's Frozen Meals**
  - **Low-sodium veggie lasagna, stuffed shells, mac and soy cheese, Mexican tamale pie, brown rice and veggie bowl, individual pizza**
  - **Any of the pockets: tofu scramble pocket (good breakfast option, Maintenance Only), feta spinach pocket**

- Breakfast Burrito (Maintenance Only)
- Toaster Pop (Maintenance Only)
- Lean Cuisine Spa Cuisine Line (more veggies)
- Healthy Choice
- Kashi
- Smart Ones
- Cedarlane
- Cedarlane Zone
- Celentano
- South Beach

VEGGIE BURGERS/MEAT-FREE PRODUCTS

In general, you should keep to the portion size listed on the package for these items. The exception is with veggie burgers as most people are not satisfied with one and really need two. This is fine if each burger is less than 120 calories. Amy's Veggie Burgers are higher in calories, so if you choose them, keep it to one burger.

- Morningstar Veggie Links
- Morningstar Veggie Burgers (can have 2)
- Morningstar Meal Starters
- Amy's Veggie Burgers (keep it to 1, these are slightly higher in calories)
- Boca Meatless Lasagna
- Boca Meatless Burgers (can have 2 at one time)
- Boca Meatless Breakfast Wrap (Maintenance Only)

Meal Replacements/Protein Powder

Any flavor.

- EAS Myoplex Lite Ready-to-Drink Shake
- EAS Myoplex Carb Sense Ready-to-Drink Shake
- EAS Myoplex Light (1 packet)
- Designer Whey Protein (1 scoop)
- Spiru-Tein (1 scoop)

Miscellaneous

- **Parchment paper**
- **Ziploc Zip 'n steam cooking bags**
- **Pyrex dishes for baking**

"When people ask me how I feel having lost so much weight, I tell them it has completely changed my life. Then they ask me how I did it and I tell them I followed the Wall Street Diet. It was easy to follow and, more importantly, I was able to stick to it. I lost fifty-nine pounds in six months and dropped six sizes. I went from size 1X to size small. One dramatic shift is that I no longer have to shop in the Plus Size department. Two friends now go to my nutritionist, Heather Bauer, and four coworkers have been so impressed by my success, they asked for Heather's phone number. People constantly tell me I am their inspiration, which makes me feel so great that I was able to accomplish this long overdue goal. I've been on maintenance for four months, and it's going well. I feel confident that I will be able to follow the Wall Street Diet for the rest of my life."

—NANCY E. WENNER, EXECUTIVE ASSISTANT, HBO

Index

fruit, 31, 50, 55–56, 98, 121, 124, 149,
  150, 153, 174, 204
  dried, 264
  portion sizes for, 64
  in power presciption breakfasts,
    176, 177
  shopping for, 306
fruit juice, 59, 139
fun snacks, 51, 61–63, 66–67, 178, 190,
  204
  shopping for, 311–12

G

gifts, food, 99–100
Gilt at the New York Palace Hotel, 231
Glaessner, Ellen, 64
goals, 83, 104, 132, 206, 209
grains, whole, 25
granola, 139
granola bars, 150, 153, 177, 311
Great Lakes Brewing Co., 271–72
Great Wraps, 264–66
Greek restaurants, 256
grooming, 212–14
gum, 160, 192
gyms, 193, 195, 197
  steam baths at, 214
  traveling and, 157, 164, 199

H

hair, 213
hamburgers, 108, 188
Happy Hour Lite, 107–8
Happy Hour Meal, 108–9, 110–11
Harnett, Mark H., 117
Hartsfield-Jackson Atlanta
  International Airport, 264–67
Heidi's Brooklyn Deli, 275
Hong Kong International Airport,
  285–86
hors d'oeuvres, 226
hotels, 160–65
  bar food at, 230–31
Houlihan's, 266

Hudson News, 150, 153, 263
hummus, 29
hunger, fatigue and, 161

I

ice cream, 49
Indian restaurants, 257
Italian restaurants, 257
iTrain, 201

J

Japanese restaurants, 257
JetBlue, 300
jet lag, 162, 163
Jody Maroni's, 272
John F. Kennedy International Airport,
  279–80
Jong, Erica, 90
journal, food, 41–43, 82–86, 198, 203–4
Journal of Labor Research, 105
Juicy Carbs, 25, 49, 50, 52–53, 54, 56
  in maintenance phase, 206–7
  plateaus and, 204
  Pleasures, 207, 208–9
  shopping for, 304–5
  soups and, 238

K

ketchup, 61
KFC, 244–45, 276
King Cole Bar & Lounge at the St.
  Regis Hotel, 230
kitchen:
  avoiding after dinner, 30, 182
  office, 96–98
KnowFat! Café, 268

L

LaGuardia Airport/New York, 281
Lauer, Kristin O., 214
Legal Sea Foods, 268–69
lentils, 52
Libassi, Thomas, 132
lifestyle, 16

turkey (*continued*)
    shopping for, 307
    as snack, 31–32, 37, 182, 190–91

U
underwear, 212–13
United Airlines, 300–303
Uno Chicago Grill, 269

V
vacations, 210–12
variety, 30
vegetables, 50, 56, 121, 153, 176
    buffets and, 140, 141
    and food safety while traveling,
        162
    as Juicy Carbs, 25, 52, 56
    shopping for, 306–7
    ten vegetable salad, 236
vegetarians, 53, 88
veggie burgers, 314
Veggie Nights, 88–89, 204
veteran dieters, 24, 39–40, 52, 53
virgin dieters, 39–40, 53
Virgin Marys, 155

W
waffles, 140, 209
walking, 200
Wall Street Diet:
    challenges in, 93–117; *see also* office
    cheat sheets for, *see* cheat sheets;
        restaurants, by name
    commute and, *see* commute
    eating out and, *see* restaurants
    exercise and, *see* exercise
    food journals in, 41–43, 82–86, 198,
        203–4
    maintenance phase of, 205–14
    meal suggestions for, 65–67
    menus for, 73–81
    nonnegotiables in, 21–22, 40
    office and, *see* office
    origins of, 15–17

personal eating ID in, 19–44; *see
    also* Clean Plate Club Eaters;
    Controlled Eaters
personal meal choices in, 70–71
plan for, 47–90
plateaus and, 202–5
preparation in, 5–6
recipes for, 68–69
recovery strategies in, 6–7, 87–89
restaurant meals and, *see*
    restaurants
setting priorities in, 4–5
shopping for, 86, 304–15
starting, 10–11
summary of, 4–7
template in, 48–64
travel and, *see* travel
vacations and, 210–12
weekend and, *see* weekends
weigh-ins and, 90, 190
Wander, the, 27–28
Wansink, Brian, 105
water, 33, 38–39, 58, 137
    air travel and, 153, 155
    Clean Plate Club eaters and, 24, 32,
        38
    commute and, 178
    office celebrations and, 95
    plateaus and, 204
    retaining, 190
    safety of, when traveling, 162
Waterworks Bar & Grill, 277
weekends, 186–201
    activity suggestions for, 193
    calorie intake on, 188–89, 192
    Fridays and, 102–4, 187–88
    kids and, 191–92
    planning ahead for, 193
    Saturdays, 188–92
    snacks on, 190–91
    Sundays, 192–93
weight:
    aftershocks and, 205
    maintenance of, 205–14